The Good Doctor

A Father, a Son, and the Evolution of Medical Ethics

BARRON H. LERNER, MD

Beacon Press
Boston

BEACON PRESS
Boston, Massachusetts
www.beacon.org

Beacon Press books
are published under the auspices of
the Unitarian Universalist Association of Congregations.

17 16 15 14   8 7 6 5 4 3 2 1

This book is printed on acid-free paper that meets the uncoated paper
ANSI/NISO specifications for permanence as revised in 1992.

Text design and composition by Kim Arney
Frontispiece photo © Barron H. Lerner

Library of Congress Cataloging-in-Publication Data

Lerner, Barron H.
The good doctor : a father, a son, and the evolution
of medical ethics / by Barron H. Lerner, MD.
    pages   cm
Includes bibliographical references.
ISBN 978-0-8070-3340-1 (hardcover : alk. paper)
ISBN 978-0-8070-3341-8 (ebook : alk. paper)
1. Lerner, Barron H. 2. Lerner, Phillip I., 1932-2012.
3. Physicians-Professional ethics. 4. Medical ethics.
5. Medical care-Decision making. I. Title.
R725.5.L47 2014
174.2—dc23
2013048242

ALSO BY BARRON H. LERNER

Contagion and Confinement: Controlling Tuberculosis along the Skid Road

The Breast Cancer Wars: Hope, Fear, and the Pursuit of a Cure in Twentieth-Century America

When Illness Goes Public: Celebrity Patients and How We Look at Medicine

One for the Road: Drunk Driving Since 1900

In loving memory of Cooper Dean Stock,
Phillip's grandson and Barron's nephew,
August 9, 2004–January 10, 2014

Contents

Prologue

The senior physician, a consultant specializing in infectious diseases, was making rounds one morning in 1996. One of his patients was a woman with end-stage vascular disease and severe arthritis that left her unable to get out of bed. Even minor changes in position caused abrasions and ulcers to form on her extremely fragile skin. The patient had been hospitalized for several months with highly resistant infections and was unlikely to ever leave. On several occasions, she had remarked to the consultant that her quality of life had become unbearable.

When the doctor and his team entered the patient's room, she was staring straight ahead and not moving. The physician checked for a pulse. There was none, but the woman's wrist was still warm. She had just died.

One of the younger physicians ran down the hall to get the patient's nurse. Hospital protocol mandated that the chest team be called and that cardiopulmonary resuscitation (CPR) be performed. Although the patient's condition was dire, her primary physician had not obtained a do-not-resuscitate (DNR) order that would have prevented the CPR.

Nevertheless, the senior physician overruled this, stating that resuscitation should not be done. But when he and his team left the ward, the nursing staff decided to call the chest team anyway. Hearing this announced on the hospital's overhead paging system, the physician returned to the bedside. That is when he did something extraordinary: he placed his body over the patient, deliberately blocking his colleagues and foiling their desperate attempts to perform CPR. Despite their frantic objections, he stayed in place for several minutes, until they finally gave up. The patient was declared dead.

Individuals who have recently spent time in hospital settings know all about DNR orders and the need for terminally ill patients to make their own end-of-life choices. This doctor's decision—to prevent the further treatment of a patient whose condition was terminal—occurred in a period of transition, when Americans were still learning about concepts like informed consent and advance directives. Nevertheless, what the senior physician did was highly irregular, violating both hospital protocol and the evolving ethical standards of the time.

This doctor's son was also a physician, trained a generation after his father. He had been studying bioethics—the very field that was establishing the new rules about death and dying. When his father told him the story, he was horrified. "You can't do that!" the shocked son cried. Of all people, he thought, how could his father, such a revered physician, so blatantly play God?

The doctor in this story is my father, Phillip I. Lerner. And I am the son.

When I was growing up, family and friends were always telling me what a wonderful doctor my father was—brilliant, a gifted teacher, and devoted to his craft. Medicine, they said, was his calling. My dad was born into a religious Jewish family in Cleveland in 1932, and his decision to become a physician stemmed from his upbringing, although he himself was not observant. He attended a medical school that emphasized a new, humanistic approach to education. Over the years, he became a highly respected infectious disease specialist, known both nationally and internationally. During my father's career, he often did not bill patients. He labored most evenings writing detailed scientific papers about cases he had encountered, spent his summer vacations in frequent phone contact with covering physicians, and rewrote his medical-school lectures every year, even though some of his colleagues couldn't be bothered to do so. He developed incredibly intense relationships with patients and families, intervening in lives, not just diseases. This type of doctoring was a dying art. But it contributed mightily to my own decision to become a physician.

After completing my residency in internal medicine in 1989, I was awarded a fellowship that enabled me to return to school to study history and bioethics. Eventually, I became one of a handful of "MD-PhD historians" who straddled the worlds of both clinical medicine and the history of medicine, seeing patients, teaching students, and writing books and articles. Much of my research into diseases like tuberculosis and breast cancer focused directly on the decisions that various physicians of my father's generation had made. Many of the ethical precepts instituted in the bioethics movement of the 1980s and 1990s, I found, came in response to transgressions made by my dad's peers in the decades after World War II.

Moreover, my father himself was one of the guilty parties. As I would learn, during his infectious diseases fellowship, he participated in experimentation on mentally disabled children without obtaining consent from the subjects or their guardians. He had a tendency to conceal information, and at times even outright lie, if he thought that such choices were in the best interests of a patient or a patient's family. And, as the above story demonstrates, he became increasingly upset—even distraught—about the use of advanced technologies to prolong the lives of dying patients, a situation that bioethicists have termed *medical futility*. On more than one occasion, my dad took matters into his own hands. Physicians, he believed, should simply not be allowed to offer aggressive options to terminally ill patients. This inclination to overrule patients and families violated the principle of patient autonomy, which was at the heart of the emergence of bioethics. Finally, my father saw little wrong in directing the medical care of his own sick relatives, an absolute taboo from our modern perspective. When I suggested that he and his colleagues had made many poor ethical judgments during their careers, he often disagreed.

Ten years after my father prevented his colleagues from administering CPR—or, as he saw it, after he permitted a terminally ill patient to die with dignity—he had developed Parkinson's disease and was cutting back on his duties as a prelude to retirement. I often visited my parents in Cleveland, and, after each trip, I returned to New York with a stack of the journals that my father had kept, with entries dating as far back as my first birthday, in September 1961.

So just what had my father been writing about so compulsively for all of those years? And why was he doing it? The earliest entries were written only annually, first on my birthdays and then, later, on my younger sister Dana's birthdays as well. They largely recounted events that had occurred during the previous year and reported on various milestones that Dana and I had reached. I was a precocious child, writing full sentences and memorizing all of the presidents well before kindergarten, which immediately suggested to my dad that I should follow in his footsteps and pursue a career in medicine. He regularly brought me to the hospital when I was a small child, even, I've been told, cloaking me in a white coat.

After a while, my father also began to write about cases on which he had served as a consultant, describing the interesting infections he had seen as well as his interactions with his patients, their families, and his colleagues. And then, in 1977, when I was sixteen years old, the floodgates opened. His journals became his primary mechanism for reflecting on two jarring events from that year: my grandfather Meyer's unexpected death and my mother's diagnosis of breast cancer at age forty-two. Like so many men of his generation, my dad was tight-lipped with his emotions and not given to outward displays of affection. But as time went on, he increasingly poured his thoughts, fears, and regrets into his journals. Reading these pages, I frequently felt like I was meeting someone I had never known. Yet the writing must have been cathartic. He would continue to confide in his journals for thirty more years. Many of his later entries remarked on how managed care, paperwork, bureaucracy, and other negative developments in medicine made him no longer love being a doctor. He wrote and wrote until 2007, when his Parkinson's disease progressed too far to allow him to produce legible and coherent sentences.

What I was learning about my father did not exactly jibe with the vaunted image of him that I had had since my childhood. Was he as wonderful a doctor as I had been told by family members, friends, and grateful patients for years? As a historian, I knew it was crucial not to evaluate the actions of past physicians using modern standards. Rather, it was necessary to use the standards of the day. His journals, many of which were written in real time, helped me to do this. So, too, a brief journal of my own, compiled when I was a third-year medical student, reminded me to place my own career in the proper historical context.

Here, then, were many important questions: How could I square my years of training in bioethics with what I now knew about my father? Was he just part of an older era of misguided—even arrogant—physicians who had lost their relevance? Or did I need to revisit the ethical norms that I had embraced and taught to thousands of medical students and residents? Moreover, how could the standards that determined an ethical physician change so drastically over only one generation? I once attended a meeting at which longtime Columbia University College of Physicians and Surgeons gastroenterologist Robert A. Whitlock called Robert F. Loeb, the legendary chair of medicine at Columbia from 1946 to 1960, "the best damned ethicist I ever met." Yet Loeb was known for bullying medical students on rounds and interacting with patients in a thoroughly domineering, albeit kind, manner. Did Whitlock's claim make any sense?

I even had to reexamine the episode in which my father covered the body of the severely ill arthritis patient. Was it possible—despite my initial revulsion—that his decision had actually been the correct one? And, more provocatively, did I wish I could have the courage to do that sort of thing myself? And what about my dad's twenty-four-hours-a-day, seven-days-a-week devotion to his profession and his patients? Was that sort of intense commitment to learning everything possible about one's patients and their diseases truly the only way to be a good doctor? Did physicians of my father's era actually know their patients in a different—and better—way than physicians do today?

There is no going back. Patients' rights are a fixture of medical practice, as they should be. The notion that doctors would deliberately conceal information from patients is almost laughable now. Concerns about sleep deprivation and family time mean that most doctors no longer spend days in a row in the hospital. Indeed, many now simply work shifts. They are as likely to be called health-care providers as physicians. Meanwhile, regulatory changes in medicine seem like a direct rebuke to my father's generation of physicians. For example, clinical guidelines now tie the hands of individual doctors, forcing them to order only cost-effective tests and to prescribe medications based on the results of randomized clinical trials as opposed to their clinical judgment. And financial concerns mandate that office visits be short and goal-directed, making it much harder for physicians to learn about patients and their families.

But reading my father's copious and detailed journal entries brought to life a seminal era in the history of medicine. Much has been gained during my time as a doctor, but much has also been lost. I came to admire many of the practices and assumptions of my dad's generation, including some that shocked me when I first learned of them. And even as the Affordable Care Act marshals scientific and economic information to reform health care in the United States, this earlier brand of medicine reminds us how the expertise and professionalism of physicians remain central to this effort.

Dr. Phillip Lerner, of course, was my parent, trying to raise me with the values that he and my mother believed in. And he was also, in a sense, in loco parentis for his sick patients, who followed his advice so they could be healed. But halfway through my father's career, those same patients—and those of his peers—began to question the doctor-as-parent model, rejecting their physicians' paternalism in favor of gaining a degree of autonomy. Meanwhile, I chose a path that honored my father's profession but also criticized it. And, at the end of his life, as my dad's Parkinson's disease worsened and therapeutic decisions needed to be made, I reluctantly took on the roles of both his doctor and his parent. In some sense, therefore, this book is about skills that are crucial for both health professionals and parents: knowing when to insist on something and knowing when to let go.

CHAPTER ONE

The First Dr. Lerner

My father's decision to become a physician stemmed from his upbringing in a close-knit, working-class Jewish community during World War II. Although he was largely unaware of the mass murder of Jews as it was occurring, what he learned later would affect many aspects of his medical world. His career trajectory was also greatly influenced by his attending a medical school that was in the forefront of efforts to train humanistic physicians. And he had an inspiring mentor who practiced a particular type of patient-centered, case-based medicine that hearkened back to the practices of some of America's greatest early doctors and reached its apogee in the mid-twentieth century.

As a historian, I was not surprised by what I read in my father's journals. After all, everyone is, to some degree, a product of his or her times. Yet as a doctor, I was amazed by much of what I read. Indeed, my dad's medical school training and early career would probably be unrecognizable to most modern physicians.

My father's story is typical for an American Jew of Ashkenazi descent whose family left Poland in the early twentieth century. Fortunately, my paternal great-grandfather, Ben Lerner, chose to immigrate to the United States as the century began. Realizing that the Jews of Poland would never belong and would never be able to live in peace, he left shortly before World War I, escaping the fate of most of the Jews of his village, Yanova: they died in the Holocaust. As was common then, he left his wife and children behind, hoping to get a foothold before sending for them. Over the years, first in Pittsburgh and then in Cleveland, Ben would work in a series of jobs, eventually running gas stations from dawn to dusk—"in good spirits," my father wrote, "because he knew what he had escaped." He was, my dad went on, a simple man with "basic values and resolve"; his favorite expression was "Hope for the best." The second-oldest child of Ben and his wife, Dora, was Meyer, my grandfather, who was born in Poland in 1907. Meyer's wife, my grandmother Pearl, was also born in Poland. Her family arrived in Cleveland in 1920. They met there in 1927 and married three years later.

Being Jewish in Cleveland at this time was all about religious commitment and unity. Both of my great-grandfathers on my father's side of the family, Ben and Chaim, belonged to the Mezricher Society, a Jewish club (or *landsmanshaft*, in Yiddish) that sponsored social events, helped welcome newcomers, and supplied cemetery plots. Chaim and his wife, Dina, were Orthodox Jews, following all the customs, such as not mixing milk and meat, not using electricity on the Sabbath, praying with phylacteries every day, and regularly going to synagogue. Ben and Dora Lerner were not as strict as Chaim and Dina, in part due to an incident in which Ben, a struggling peddler at the time, was turned away from High Holiday services at a temple because he could not afford a ticket. Thanks to Dora, however, they still observed most of the religious rituals. Yiddish was the mother tongue in both homes, although the families spoke more and more English over time.

By the 1920s, Cleveland's Jewish community had mostly congregated on the city's east side, in an area known as Glenville. The main thoroughfare was East 105th Street, which, one historian wrote, was "lined with Jewish bakeries, pharmacies, shops and important charitable and religious institutions." There were still peddlers with horse-drawn wagons. Life centered on the family. My father had eighteen first cousins, several of whom lived in a two-family house on Eddy Road that the Lerners shared with one of Pearl's sisters and her family. His cousins were his best friends, and with so many relatives living within a few blocks, informal socializing on the stoops of houses or in local playgrounds was the rule.

My grandfather Meyer worked steadily as a furrier during the 1930s and 1940s, despite the Great Depression and the deprivations of World War II. Although I always knew that these events had shaped my father's life, his journals revealed just how directly his family, class, and religion affected his eventual career choice. His parents expected him to earn money during high school, and he did. They also expected him to succeed in ways that they, as first-generation immigrants from the working class, could not. College was an absolute certainty. During college, my dad worked in his father's fur shop as well as in the local butcher shop. In medical school, he drove a creaky electric trolley bus with straw mesh seats for the old Cleveland Transit System in some of the most dangerous parts of town. "Love of family, honesty and hard work," he wrote many years later, were the "common values of strong families in those days."

The fact that my dad was a diligent and enthusiastic student surely helped him achieve his goals. In later years, he would characterize his youth as mundane and his view of the world beyond Cleveland as completely naïve. Before visiting St. Louis, New York, Boston and other cities in 1958 at age twenty-five to interview for a medical residency, he had never been so far from home. The only real vacations that the family had taken were trips to Pittsburgh to see relatives. But his experiences in Cleveland, working hard to help support his family while also excelling in school, prepared him to move beyond the confines of his provincial upbringing.

He chose medicine as a career not only because it was a path to the middle class but also because of his experiences growing up Jewish in the 1930s and 1940s. He attended Glenville High School, a predominantly Jewish public school filled with second-generation-immigrant teenagers from working-class families with lofty aspirations. The informal name for Glenville students, the Tarblooders, came from a local tar company and reflected how hard these children were willing to work at school and sports in order to succeed. Brooklyn and the Grand Concourse in the Bronx are the repositories for memories of New York Jewish children coming of age in the mid-twentieth century, and Glenville and its high school serve the same role for Clevelanders. Still, after his Orthodox bar mitzvah, my father concluded that religion meant little to him. Mild-mannered Meyer, who took enormous pride in his sons' accomplishments, often let my dad and his younger brother, Allan, know that he was nonetheless disappointed that they had turned their backs on their faith.

But they really had not. Even though my father would resist going to temple for decades, his identity as a Jew and the moral teachings he encountered in Hebrew school stuck with him. As the writer Abigail Pogrebin has detailed, this generation of Jews "absorbed a sense of peril, the need to prove themselves [and the need] to stay connected to the Jewish community." Learning about that existential peril, the Holocaust, affected my dad's outlook profoundly. When World War II ended, media reports—and the arrival in America of distant cousins of his who had survived concentration camps—brought home the full scale of the horror. "Growing up in this magic country and peacefully going to school, smothered and protected by my family and the circumstances of the times," my father wrote, he had not known of any of the atrocities that were going on in Europe. He realized, as he later put it, that he had been "spared by one generation" from almost certain death. "It was your great-great-grandfather Ben Lerner," he wrote in a journal entry addressed to my son, also named Ben Lerner, on the day of his birth in 1993, whose "adventurous spirit and gutsy determination" had "made our lives possible" by sparing the family from the deprivation, danger, and doom experienced by Jews in Europe during the 1930s and 1940s.

More subtly, surviving the Holocaust in the safety of the United States helped forge my father's career path. It stood to reason that with such an acute sense of survivor's guilt and an appreciation for his good luck, my dad would choose a profession that first and foremost enabled him to help others. And he would become a physician who was fiercely devoted to his patients, more than a few of whom were themselves Holocaust survivors.

As with many teenagers who aspire to be physicians, my father had a role model. In the era of the house call, a dedicated Cleveland general practitioner named Clarence Weidenthal was a regular visitor at all hours to the house on Eddy Road. In his journals, my dad recalled an incident when—in his late teens—he ran into Weidenthal somewhere in Cleveland. It had been at least five years since they had seen each other but, according to my father, "after a few minutes of mental gymnastics, [he] offered not only my family name, but the address, and the street, and that I had lived in one of the two suites in a 2-family home on Eddy Road." That sort of intimate knowledge of one's patients made a lasting impression.

There was little doubt that my father would attend Adelbert, the undergraduate college of Western Reserve University, located in downtown Cleveland's University Circle, home to many of the city's cultural institutions. He received a partial scholarship and offset the remaining tuition costs by living at home and continuing to work. He remained in Cleveland for medical school, enrolling in 1954 at the Western Reserve University School of Medicine (the merger of Western Reserve University and the Case Institute of Technology would occur in 1967).

It was an exciting and dynamic time to be at Western Reserve. The vast majority of medical schools in this era taught in a very traditional manner. The first two years consisted of classroom lectures and laboratories. Students spent years three and four on the wards, essentially as clinical clerks, learning from residents and attending physicians and caring for patients for the first time. By and large, a mid-twentieth-century medical school education was rote and dull.

But in 1952, three of Western Reserve's faculty members banded together to revolutionize and humanize the curriculum: Dean Joseph T. Wearn, Director of Admissions John L. "Cactus Jack" Caughey Jr., and a dapper hematologist with the memorable name of T. Hale Ham. Their idea was to turn students into "colleagues," inspiring them to do independent research and introducing them to patient care in their first year. In addition, rather than requiring separate courses in traditional subjects like biochemistry, pathology, and physiology, the Western Reserve educators reconfigured instruction to focus on specific organ systems. Professors from multiple departments worked together to integrate their information into a more dynamic whole. At the beginning of medical school, each first-year student was assigned a pregnant woman to follow, and the student was expected to care for her through and after the birthing process, even making home visits. Focus on the patient as a person was key, as was getting to know one's patients' families. (Western Reserve was farsighted, but only to a point. Only nine of the seventy-eight students in my father's class were women. And both professors and students smoked during lectures, even those lectures about cancer.)

The gruff, "bullet-shaped" Caughey prided himself on accepting nontraditional medical students, such as those who were older and had had other careers, if he believed they were especially interesting or focused on the humanistic aspects of medicine. My father's classmates included H. Jack Geiger, who would later help found both Physicians for Human Rights and Physicians for Social Responsibility; Abraham B. Bergman, a pediatrician and public health pioneer who championed the use of bicycle helmets for children; and Sadja Stokowski, daughter of conductor Leopold Stokowski, who became an early advocate for abortion rights. And my dad's faculty preceptor, who supervised his first-year clinical work, was Benjamin Spock, the legendary pediatrician and author of the best-selling 1946 book *Baby and Child Care*.

A star student, my father quickly realized that he'd made the right decision in attending medical school. He was endlessly fascinated with both the scientific explanations of diseases and the personal stories of people who were sick. He graduated near the top of his class, and Western Reserve would have been happy to have him remain in Cleveland for his internship and residency in internal medicine. But my dad knew that his academic performance placed him in high demand everywhere, and he decided it was time to look beyond Cleveland.

So the young man who had traveled so little took the train to St. Louis to interview at the renowned Barnes Hospital of Washington University. The University of Rochester and the Yale–New Haven Hospital were also on his list. In New York, he interviewed at

Bellevue Hospital, New York Hospital, and Columbia-Presbyterian Medical Center. At Columbia he met with Robert Loeb, the chairman of the Department of Medicine and the coeditor of the famous Cecil-Loeb *Textbook of Medicine*. My father's most vivid memory of his interviews is jarring but says a lot about the enormous egos of medical school professors of the era. During one interview, held in a laboratory, the physician calmly stood up and urinated into a sink, continuing to speak the whole time. My dad assumed it was some sort of test, but he was not impressed.

In Boston, he interviewed at Beth Israel Hospital, which had been founded in 1916 to serve a growing Jewish immigrant population who spoke primarily Yiddish and who kept kosher. By the mid-twentieth century, Jewish hospitals in Boston and elsewhere had opened their doors to a broad range of patients, and Beth Israel had become affiliated with Harvard. But these hospitals also served an unintended role: training Jewish medical students and residents who were excluded from Yale, Cornell, Columbia, and other prestigious hospitals that had secret quotas limiting the number of Jews. My father did not think he wound up at Beth Israel due to quotas elsewhere, but the hospital's Jewish heritage made it a comfortable home away from home.

Today, residency interviews usually involve a thirty-minute chat with a single professor and only an occasional probing question. In the 1950s, however, would-be residents were grilled by committees of doctors, who assessed each young physician's clinical knowledge and ability to think on his feet under pressure. For my father, a strong interview at Beth Israel and a supportive letter from T. Hale Ham, who had formerly been at Harvard, did the trick. In July 1958, the quiet, studious boy from Cleveland began his internal medicine residency at the famed B.I., as it was known—a "miraculous coup," he wrote many years later. Of the nine other interns admitted to the internal medicine program, seven had come from Harvard Medical School, one from Cornell, and one from the University of Chicago. Western Reserve sent almost no students to Boston.

Residents are also known as house officers or house staff. In this case, the house is the hospital, which, in the 1950s, essentially served as a home for those training in medicine. Residents were on call as often as every other night. Many, like my father, lived in rooms either in or adjacent to the hospital, which provided easy access to work. The arrangement was a quid pro quo. In exchange for staffing teaching hospitals for countless hours at very low salaries, young physicians received top-notch training from renowned professors. They were also given tremendous autonomy in the care of nonpaying patients, who were at times callously termed *teaching material* and who often spent their hospital stays in large, multi-bed wards.

Fittingly, perhaps, many residency programs had explicit or implicit rules stating that residents—who were overwhelmingly men—could not be married. Spouses were seen as too distracting for physicians working long hours and weekends. Thus, it was completely unexpected when, in November 1958, my father eloped.

My mother, Ronnie, was a native New Yorker, born in Brooklyn in 1934 to Emanuel (Mannie) and Jessie Hober. Mannie, born in New York in 1901, was a real character. As a young man, he had been both a pool shark and an amateur boxer, claiming, perhaps apocryphally, to have sparred with the great Jewish lightweight Benny Leonard. During my childhood years, Mannie worked in a hat factory. Jessie, born in Poland in 1907, raised my mother and her older brother, Mark, and later worked in a women's clothing store. When my mother was nine, the family moved to Framingham, Massachusetts, where my mother completed high school, after which she matriculated at the University of Massachusetts in Amherst. Interestingly, by moving to Framingham in the 1940s, my grandparents became a part of medical history. Both Mannie and Jessie were enrolled in the famous Framingham Heart Study, which eventually proved that high blood pressure, smoking, diabetes, and high cholesterol were related to the development of heart disease.

When my mother and father met, she had graduated from college and was a first-grade teacher. As usual, my dad ruminated on the role of fate when he thought of their marriage, which he called a "crazy miracle": My father had been perusing the little black book of a fellow intern, who was a bit of a playboy, and he asked if he could call one of the women. The intern said yes, and my father randomly chose my mother. They went on a few dates, and at times, she would come over to Beth Israel at 10 p.m., when my father and the other house officers had a snack break. But my mom, beautiful and popular, had several other boyfriends.

One day, my very opinionated grandmother Jessie announced that she'd read in the newspaper's horoscope section that it was time for Geminis to settle down. A Gemini, and ever the dutiful daughter, my mother contemplated which of her beaus would make the most suitable husband, and then, with Jessie's approval, she chose my father. Prior to getting engaged, they had spent fewer than forty hours together. It was only years later that Jessie admitted she had made up the whole horoscope story.

The decision to elope stunned both families. The honeymoon itself, in New Hampshire, lasted all of two days and occurred only because a fellow intern volunteered to cover for my father. For my mother, it was a sign of things to come. For years, work would always come first for Dr. Lerner.

As one would expect, there were many luminaries at the Beth Israel. The chair of medicine from 1928 to 1962 was Hermann Blumgart, the first physician to measure blood flow and to inject a radioactive tracer into the blood for diagnostic purposes. Also on staff was Paul M. Zoll, a cardiologist who developed the first functional external cardiac pacemaker. But my father's favorite attending physician was Louis Zetzel, a gastroenterologist who had originally intended to become a rabbi and who continued to make house calls until he was seventy-seven years old. "My idea of what a family physician should be," Zetzel once said, "means his availability to his patients, even if this entails the inconveniences and interruptions of his private life."

The 1950s has been called the golden age of medicine, as physicians, armed with a remarkable series of new treatments, saved or extended the lives of those who surely would have died only a couple of decades earlier. Integral to this perception was a fierce devotion to the science and scientific research that had contributed to these recent triumphs. "What's new in *Wissenschaft*?" asked

Columbia-Presbyterian's Robert Loeb when interested house officers, students, and faculty members crowded into his small office at
7 a.m. for a daily informal discussion of developments in medicine.

Perhaps the most iconic image of this era is that of a large group
of physicians decked out in their white coats surrounding a patient.
At most hospitals, these doctors were by and large white and male.
At times, a patient's nurse—a woman—stood quietly near the revered group. Generally such rounds were led by a senior professor;
the crowd included medical residents, medical students, and visiting
physicians spending the day at the institution. Much ink has been
spilled on the significance of the white coat. Although the phalanx of
white may have inspired confidence in worried patients, it is surely
also true that such rounds could be intimidating.

At Columbia, Loeb, who rounded seven days a week, was known
for his fanatical devotion to all the patients—rich and poor—on
the medical service. Being a doctor, he believed, meant knowing
every last detail of their medical histories and their lives. Loeb
imparted this philosophy to decades of trainees. A quote posted
on the wall of Columbia's Department of Medicine, attributed to
internist and future Nobel Prize winner Dickinson Richards Jr.,
summed up this attitude: "Who is responsible for this patient and
where the hell is he at?" This demand for excellence extended to
medical students, who Loeb relentlessly grilled when he believed
they had not adequately prepared. On more than one occasion, patients actually upbraided Loeb for being too tough on their "doctors." Sure, Loeb was a martinet, Columbia cardiologist William
Lovejoy once told me, but why shouldn't he have been one? Patient care was "life or death."

The opportunity to learn from great professors inspired generations of physicians. In my book on the history of breast cancer, I
wrote about how William S. Halsted of the Johns Hopkins School
of Medicine set up the first surgical residency program, training a
group of surgeons who then became professors at hospitals across
the country and who, in turn, mentored their own trainees. In this
manner, it was possible to trace generations of surgeons back to Halsted. This kind of connection had many virtues, such as ensuring

that important skills and knowledge were passed down, although, in the case of breast cancer, it also had the unfortunate consequence of ensuring that Halsted's disfiguring radical mastectomy operation was used for far too long.

My father found his own mentor in his second year, when he was doing a hematology rotation at the New England Medical Center, Tufts University School of Medicine's teaching hospital. With an hour to kill one day, he attended a lecture on meningococcemia, a severe blood infection, given by Louis Weinstein. Years later, my dad recalled having been "transfixed" at the precision and detail of Weinstein's presentation. He had found, "by an incredible stroke of good fortune, the proper niche for my medical talents and teaching-research instincts, by falling under the spell of a mesmerizing, dynamic teacher who is fanatic, encyclopedic, opinionated, scholarly and demanding of his specialty and all those who aspire to it or intersect its vast boundaries."

Weinstein typically spoke without notes or slides for an hour or more, peppering his lectures with memorable cases from his own career. He was a great storyteller. After the lecture, my father introduced himself to Weinstein and rather boldly asked if he needed an infectious diseases fellow one year later, when my dad completed his residency. Coincidentally, a spot had just opened up in Weinstein's program.

But was my father the right person for the position? In his papers, I found a letter of recommendation written on onionskin paper by the chief physician at Beth Israel terming him an "outstanding" resident who was "well above average in professional capacity." Even more important than the recommendation, however, was the old-boys network so prevalent in medicine in this era. Weinstein, it turned out, was good friends with Samuel Lewis, a Beth Israel neurosurgeon. As fate would have it, my dad had recently gone above and beyond with one of Lewis's brain tumor patients, staying up all night with him. When Weinstein called Lewis for the scoop, the deal was done. It was telling to read this anecdote a half century after it occurred; new work-hour rules that truncate hospital shifts might well have prohibited what my father did.

Weinstein was truly one of the pioneers of the field of infectious diseases, "a bridge between the eras before and after the introduction of antibiotics," according to one of his colleagues. Since Weinstein had trained as a microbiologist before becoming an internist, it would have made sense for him to go on to specialize in infectious diseases—but the field did not yet exist. However, there were still isolation hospitals for people with contagious and communicable diseases, and in the late 1940s and early 1950s, he ran one of them, the John C. Haynes Memorial Hospital, located just outside of Boston. Like the superintendents of the old sanatoriums for tuberculosis, Weinstein lived on the grounds of the Haynes with his wife and children.

It was at the Haynes that Weinstein became a great diagnostician, the skill that made him legendary and most attracted my father. There, Weinstein treated epidemics of several infectious diseases, including scarlet fever, pertussis (whooping cough) and diphtheria. In the case of diphtheria, which had been brought to Boston by soldiers returning from Germany in the late 1940s, Weinstein admitted many children whose physicians had missed the classic sign of the disease, the characteristic thick, yellow membrane coating the throat; those physicians had mistakenly diagnosed strep and prescribed penicillin, which is ineffective for diphtheria. But it was during two polio outbreaks—in 1949 and 1955—that Weinstein really made his mark, often starting rounds at six in the morning and not finishing until midnight. Among the polio patients he treated were four pregnant women who required ventilation with iron lungs. Despite several attempts, he was unable to get any Boston obstetricians to deliver the babies due to their fear of contagion. Fortunately, when Weinstein was a Boston University medical student on call at Boston City Hospital years earlier, he had fetched sodas and magazines for obstetrics residents in exchange for being allowed to deliver babies. So Weinstein himself successfully delivered the four babies—"one-handed," he liked to brag—as he could not fit both of his hands into the tight confines of the iron lung.

By the mid-1950s, contagious diseases were on the decline. Among the reasons for this development was the growing number of antibiotics available—not only penicillin but the sulfonamides, streptomycin, and isoniazid for tuberculosis. Weinstein was one of many of his generation to witness miraculous cures: in the late 1940s, he saw a moribund girl with meningitis recover completely when given streptomycin. Previously fatal infections, such as pneumonia and sepsis, could now be conquered. As my father often remarked, these dramatic cures were one of the greatest appeals of the specialty eventually called infectious diseases. Other than surgery, there were few interventions in medicine that could so drastically improve the condition of a patient with a serious disease. There seemed to be no limit to what scientific research could achieve.

When it was time for Weinstein to leave the Haynes, he moved to Tufts and the New England Medical Center to continue his work, positioning himself as an expert on both infections and the choice of antibiotics. It was the birth of infectious diseases as a specialty, and when my father completed his internal medicine residency, in 1961, he continued his career as a fellow under Louis Weinstein. By this time, there was another Dr. Lerner on the scene—at least a future one. I had been born in September 1960.

In order to better demonstrate the type of medicine my father practiced and what a career in medicine meant to him, one can create a genealogy similar to that of Halsted and his trainees. The best place to start is with Halsted's Johns Hopkins colleague William Osler, who was the world's best-known internist in the late nineteenth and early twentieth centuries. At the time, the majority of physicians were generalists—comfortable treating most medical conditions—but Osler's knowledge was unparalleled, as witnessed by his authorship of one of the era's definitive textbooks, *The Principles and Practice of Medicine*. Osler was also an exceptional teacher who helped to revolutionize the Johns Hopkins School of Medicine and, as a result, medical school education. Finally, Osler was a great humanist, and he worried that specialization and overreliance on drugs could deleteriously deflect the attention of the medical profession away from patients. "The good physician treats the disease," he wrote. "The great physician treats the patient who has the disease."

Among the small-town general practitioners who swore by the Osler text was John B. Beeson, who saw patients in Montana, Washington, Alaska, and Ohio between 1904 and 1957, when he retired at age eighty-five. One of Beeson's two physician sons was Paul B. Beeson, and he kept Osler's spirit alive through decades as a researcher, professor, and later dean of the Yale School of Medicine. Beeson did pathbreaking research on endocarditis, hepatitis, and fevers of unknown origin. He became a coeditor of the Cecil-Loeb textbook of medicine, which eventually supplanted the Osler volume, and later in his career moved to Oxford University, as had Osler. He trained large numbers of medical students and residents through his teaching rounds on the wards. But Beeson most resembled Osler in his humanism—his "quiet attention to each individual patient" and his "powerful sense of caring."

In 1939 and 1940, Beeson had been chief medical resident at Harvard's Peter Bent Brigham Hospital, serving under another famed physician-teacher, Soma Weiss. Weiss, in turn, had been a colleague of Chester Keefer, Louis Weinstein's mentor. So when my father joined Weinstein as a fellow, he could trace his medical lineage back to Keefer, Weiss, Beeson, and finally Osler.

Although I did find a reprint of a 1980 article, "What's So Special about Osler?," in my dad's papers, he would not have formally considered himself an Oslerian. But my father followed in the footsteps of those physicians who were comfortable with any type of medical problem, who taught young doctors with great passion, and who believed that connecting emotionally with patients was the greatest success they could have. And while they rarely took no for an answer from either colleagues or patients, these physicians viewed their decisions as being in the best interests of their patients. To complete the circle, when I did a fellowship in Seattle, I had lunch on a few occasions with the affable Paul Beeson, who had returned from England and become a distinguished professor at the University of Washington.

In recounting my father's fellowship, I find it hard not to think of the excitement and optimism of the early 1960s. As the space program, the War on Poverty, and the civil rights movement unfolded, my father and his peers were expanding the study of antibiotics in the laboratory, publishing groundbreaking scientific research, bringing their findings to the bedsides of acutely ill patients, and saving lives that might have been lost just a decade before. And Weinstein was a great mentor. To be sure, Weinstein could be brusque and had a healthy ego; one of his trainees later wrote a satirical book, *Heartsblood*, that was quite critical of the revered professors of this era. But Weinstein saw things that others missed. His personal clinical knowledge—acquired through decades of hands-on experience with infected patients—was undeniable and inspiring. In 1962, for example, Weinstein diagnosed a case of typhoid fever in a man with a mass in his neck. The rest of the patient's doctors believed the man had cancer. In another instance, when consulting on a physician's child, Weinstein diagnosed whooping cough, which he had frequently seen at the Haynes; several other physicians had missed the distinctive *whoop* sound. Eventually, he instituted combined rounds, at which infectious diseases cases were presented at various hospitals in Boston in front of fellows, residents, students, and distinguished visitors.

In addition to teaching diagnostic skills to his fellows, Weinstein closely supervised them outside the hospital. At his Monday-evening journal club, an informal gathering of roughly fifteen physicians held in his West Newton home, Weinstein would lead discussions of the latest discoveries about infections and antibiotics as his fellows enjoyed brownies and, almost to a man, smoked cigarettes. This interaction—debating the scientific literature and how it might improve the treatment of patients—was the crux of the fellowship experience, the intellectual hook that had brought these young physicians together. When a fellow missed a meeting, Weinstein called him the next day for an explanation. "I do miss those old journal clubs on the ping pong table," my father's former colleague Kenneth Kaplan wrote to him in 1977, "with the paralyzing clouds of smoke, while Hardy nodded in the corner and the dog barked upstairs and the boss barked downstairs."

This collegial atmosphere, with its emphasis on applied research, ultimately led to my father's coauthoring nine peer-reviewed articles with Weinstein. The first, published in July 1964, looked at how well penicillin and a popular sulfa drug were absorbed in the intestines of diabetic patients. Another compared the effectiveness of penicillin versus a newer class of antibiotics, known as cephalosporins, in the treatment of certain bacterial infections. My dad was the first author on these papers; most mentors—including Weinstein—rarely permitted this, especially with a first paper.

But it was a four-part series by Lerner and Weinstein in the prestigious *New England Journal of Medicine* in early 1966 that suddenly accelerated my father's career. Entitled "Infective Endocarditis in the Antibiotic Era," the articles used one hundred cases of that disease treated at the New England Medical Center to summarize the dramatic changes that had occurred in the previous ten years. The choice of the word *infective*, as opposed to *bacterial*, was a conscious one, reminding readers that multiple types of organisms could infect heart valves. Other physicians readily embraced the new terminology. The phrase *antibiotic era* was also a conscious decision, meant to underscore how antimicrobial agents had transformed— almost magically—an incurable disease into a treatable one. While researching these papers, my father had spoken with the famous Harvard cardiologist Samuel A. Levine, who had told him that, prior to antibiotics, desperate doctors had actually injected dying endocarditis patients with even more dangerous bacteria, hoping to somehow increase the patients' immune responses to their original infections.

Despite his own longtime interest in endocarditis and his senior position, Weinstein again let my father, who had done most of the legwork, be listed as first author on the four articles. This was quite a coup for a thirty-three-year-old assistant professor of medicine. Because there were four separate articles, the authors were able to cover nearly every topic related to endocarditis, including the organisms that caused it, the choice of antibiotics, the role of surgery, complications, prognosis, and prevention. The series became the definitive summary of endocarditis for years, perhaps even decades. Much later, when I was a medical resident and beginning to write my own articles, my dad told me with rare self-satisfaction that his series on endocarditis was among the one hundred most cited articles in the history of the *New England Journal.*

But my father was growing restless at Tufts, frustrated by the huge time commitment and the relatively low financial rewards of a career in academic medicine. Even as the *New England Journal* series was being published, he was looking for jobs elsewhere. Weinstein was upset, practically offering him his own job once he retired. But my dad did not see himself running a laboratory or administering a fellowship program. When the Veterans Administration hospital in his hometown of Cleveland offered him a position, he took it. Weinstein was sure he'd be back, telling him, "You'll have my job someday."

Another person dissatisfied with my father's decision was my mother. Having grown up in Brooklyn and then the Boston suburbs, where her parents still lived, she had been unimpressed with Cleveland on her several visits there. But in those days, nonworking wives did not get a vote. My dad dispatched her to Cleveland to look for a house, and, in 1966, our branch of the Lerner family returned to Ohio. I was five years old and about to start first grade. My father's Cleveland relatives were excited that the studious and earnest boy who had become the first physician in the family was returning home. But he would find that the close-knit group of cousins from his youth had dispersed around the suburbs.

My father adjusted quickly to his new position as chief of infectious diseases at the VA and assistant professor at what would soon be known as the Case Western University School of Medicine. He also offered his services as an infectious diseases consultant at other Cleveland hospitals. This arrangement not only supplemented his income but allowed him to see an ongoing stream of great cases, something that he had found so rewarding in Boston.

Working at a government hospital had its challenges. In his home office, my father hung a cartoon of a Civil War soldier with an arrow through his arm patiently sitting in a VA waiting room, still hoping to be seen by a doctor a hundred years after his injury. But as a child, I loved to visit the hospital, where my dad was always being paged on the overhead PA system, which thrilled me even more than the parking space with his name on it. I remember the floors with multiple-colored arrows directing visitors and staff members to the X-ray department, the cafeteria, and other parts of the hospital.

I spent much of every Saturday with my father. When I was still quite young, my mother enrolled me in music-theory classes and piano lessons at the Cleveland Music School Settlement, also located in University Circle. Typically, my dad would drop me off at my lessons and pick me up a couple of hours later. Sometimes, we went out to lunch. Other times, especially when I was younger, we went back to the hospital, where he would bring me onto the wards and plop me in the nurses' station while he made rounds. Whether or not the legend of my wearing a white coat during such visits was true, the nurses and other staff members always made a big deal out of my being there. My father brought my sister to the hospital as well, but he was not nearly as focused on her becoming a doctor. Perhaps this was because she was a girl in an era in which most doctors were still men, but it also may have reflected the fact that she did not really enjoy math and science.

Another frequent stop was the microbiology laboratory. To this day, I can remember the distinctive sanitized odor of the lab. The technicians always greeted my father warmly, perhaps because he was one of the few doctors who knew them all by name and who looked for bacteria himself, putting infectious material on a slide and staining it—creating what is known as a Gram stain. This was a major issue for my dad, who feared that internists were becoming too reliant on technicians and specialists when it came to the diagnostic studies—not only slides but X-rays and biopsies—performed on their patients. Even so, he made a point of praising lab technicians who did a good job. And he showed me how to grow bacteria on agar plates and how to test them against various antibiotic agents—an early introduction to laboratory technique that fascinated me. "Plate your own cultures" was his chronic refrain to younger doctors.

No topic was more important to my father than hand-washing. Some men's heroes are athletes, actors, or politicians. My dad's was the heretical nineteenth-century physician Ignaz Semmelweis who was born in Budapest, Hungary, in 1818. As a young obstetrician in

Vienna, Semmelweis made the initially counterintuitive observation that at his hospital, women whose babies were delivered by medical students or physicians died of puerperal (or childbed) fever at a far higher rate following childbirth than women whose babies were delivered by midwives. Noting that the students and doctors often performed autopsies prior to attending births, he deduced that they were inadvertently transmitting an unknown "cadaverous material" that caused puerperal fever in the healthy women. Semmelweis then set up an experiment in which he required those who performed autopsies to thoroughly wash their hands with a chlorinated lime solution prior to the performance of internal examinations. When the death rate fell to that found on the other ward, he believed that he had proven his case. Once the germ theory of disease was elucidated in the late nineteenth century, the rest of the world would agree.

It was easy to see why my father, as an infectious diseases specialist, was obsessed with hand-washing, which, in the 1960s and 1970s, occurred at a disturbingly low rate in hospitals. I was probably the only teenager of my era to read cover to cover *The Cry and the Covenant*, a fictionalized version of Semmelweis's career. Sadly, things ended badly for him, as he became increasingly dogmatic and mentally ill in his later years. Little did I know at the time that these unfortunate aspects of Semmelweis's life would to some degree mirror what would happen with my dad.

I was a smart kid, and by fourth grade, my parents had moved me out of public school and into Hawken School, an all-boys private institution. It was difficult for my father not to envision me as the next Dr. Lerner. When I was in my teens, he no longer took me to the nurses' station while he made rounds but instead brought me to his Saturday medical school lectures. These occurred mostly in the late spring, when the infectious diseases committee, of which he was the de facto head, lectured the second-year medical students. I remember feeling proud, but also bored. I was a good science student but not one of those kids fascinated by how the human body works—or malfunctions. The medical students, however, paid close attention to my dad's well-received lectures, which he never delivered from prepared notes. Instead, he showed slides, told stories, and shared cases. He cared deeply about his lectures and liked to reward the students who chose to attend these classes.

An annual highlight was the committee's first lecture, when my father brought to class a rather disgusting but certainly vivid example of pus. What better way to introduce medical students to infections than by showing them what a really bad one could produce? Years before, instead of disposing of the contents of a large empyema (infected chest cavity), he had saved the material in a jar. Between its annual appearances, the jar stayed in our garage. Later in my life, when a former Case Western Reserve medical student realized that I was Phil Lerner's son, his or her next words were often: "Jar of pus!"

The only pictures that remain from my father's time at the VA are, ironically, of his going-away party in 1973. I was thirteen, and in the photos, I look like I do not want to be there at all. Given the reasons my dad became a doctor, his shift to the Mount Sinai Hospital, another teaching affiliate of Case Western, was a logical one. Mount Sinai had a history similar to that of Beth Israel in Boston: it had been built in 1913 to serve Cleveland's immigrant Jews. But by the 1970s, African Americans had largely replaced the Jewish residents who—like my father—had once lived in the neighborhood around the hospital, and Mount Sinai now served both groups. Treating this new inner-city minority population plus Jews who had moved to the suburbs was just the right mix for my dad—a doctor who viewed illness as inseparable from the details of patients' lives. The Mount Sinai was appealing for one other reason: his younger brother, Allan, who had also become a physician, was an interventional radiologist on staff there.

Louis Weinstein was certain that my father's career had peaked when he was in Boston and declined once he left for the hinterlands of Cleveland. But in the 1970s, ensconced at Mount Sinai, where he was one of Cleveland's best-known infectious diseases specialists, a well-regarded junior professor at Case Western, and, in his spare time, a clinical researcher, my dad was at the top of his game. Moreover, having crafted a job that gave him considerable autonomy and professional satisfaction, he was blissfully happy.

CHAPTER TWO

Super Doctor

I have written several books on the history of medicine, and I readily admit to having had unrealistic expectations about how many copies of each would be bought. Tuberculosis, breast cancer, and even celebrity patients were less compelling topics than I had anticipated. Still, I had to chuckle when I read of my father's onetime plan to publish a book entitled *Consultant*, detailing his experiences seeing patients with infectious diseases at the Veterans Administration Hospital, Mount Sinai Hospital, and other Cleveland medical institutions in the 1960s and 1970s. As my agent could have told him, the subject was too "specialized."

Fortunately, however, my father saved his notes, which not only illuminate his early medical career but also provide a moving depiction of him at the height of his powers, as he was practicing an intense type of medicine that might best be described as all-consuming. My dad provided a crucial service to internists, surgeons, and other physicians by diagnosing the illnesses of their sick patients and then prescribing effective antibiotics. His overarching concern for the physician-patient relationship also shone through in many of the cases that he documented

As an infectious diseases consultant, my father turned out to have a front-row seat to some of the emerging ethical issues—such as medical errors and the limits of medical technology—that would soon burst forth into the public spotlight. But his approach to these issues remained largely based on paternalism and beneficence: How could and should the doctor help his patient navigate these complicated and often controversial questions? Given his background and training, which stressed "Doctor knows best," he could hardly have chosen a different approach.

Meanwhile, I was a fairly typical teenager, trying to balance schoolwork, friends, and jobs. Two important decisions I made during these years were to have a bar mitzvah and to work for two summers at a nursing home at which my father was the medical director. The first represented an important exploration of my Judaism, although, like my father, I had great ambivalence about religion. The second turned out to be a dry run for my becoming a doctor.

Not all cases of infection require an infectious diseases consultation. Garden-variety pneumonias and urinary tract infections, for example, can be treated with a standard assortment of antibiotics. The task becomes even easier if a culture of the infectious material—such as sputum, urine, or blood—grows a specific organism. The microbiology laboratory can then test specific drugs against the bacteria in question, simplifying the choice of medication.

So when my dad was called in on a case, it was a good bet that it was complicated, either because the source of infection could not be determined or because the choice of antibiotic was unclear. For the most part, my father was happy with this arrangement. Like most physicians, he loved difficult and unusual cases, as they made for interesting discussions in the hospital corridors, on rounds, and at the citywide infectious diseases conferences he inaugurated in Cleveland in the late 1960s. Plus, even though my dad was incredibly busy, being a consultant provided him with considerably more flexibility and independence than his colleagues had, with their regular office hours and hundreds, perhaps thousands, of patients.

A typical case that my father saw in the early 1970s was a man with a lymphoma and an unusual pneumonia whose doctors were deciding whether or not to do a lung biopsy, which would involve opening the man's chest. Deducing that the man had pneumocystis pneumonia, which occurred in immunosuppressed patients and would later become a common malady of the AIDS era, he convinced the team to skip the biopsy and treat the patient empirically with antibiotics. The man recovered completely.

So did a teenager with congenital heart disease who had endocarditis. Despite being treated with penicillin, he was still running temperatures as high as 105. The patient's cardiologist was worried because the infection was not getting better, and he consulted a surgeon about replacing the infected heart valve—a major operation that the boy might not have survived. Noting that, despite his high temperature, the patient appeared to be improving, my father implored the physicians to hold off on surgery. He added another antimicrobial agent to treat what he thought was a small pneumonia. The patient never required surgery and was cured of both infections.

A man with pancreatic cancer had recurrent bacterial blood infections. He had recently become infected with a highly resistant strain of an organism called *Serratia*. The team was at a loss as to what to do to save the man's life. My father reached into his bag of tricks and suggested trying an older antibiotic, tetracycline, not normally used for this type of blood infection. The patient recovered, although he ultimately died from the cancer.

When an eighty-five-year-old man was admitted to the hospital with a severe infection of his neck, my father was able to diagnose a condition that was very rare: Ludwig's phlegmon. The infection, which had first been described by German physician Wilhelm Frederick von Ludwig in 1836, had become uncommon in the antimicrobial era but was still featured in infectious diseases textbooks. The infection required drainage of the abscess in the operating room, and my dad scrubbed in for the procedure. The surgeon had so little experience with such cases that he took my father's recommendation that he do an extra-long "guillotine incision" of the neck to help treat the patient.

My dad's consult notes, which reflected his intimate knowledge of the diseases in question, were often tutorials for the doctors (and patients) involved. When an elderly man with advanced lung disease continued to have fevers and positive sputum cultures, my father wrote: "In patients with chronic restrictive pulmonary disease, who have trouble raising secretions, antibiotic therapy of an acute pulmonary infection leads to bacterial overgrowth of the respiratory secretions." The treatment: stop antibiotics and pound on the man's back four times daily to mobilize his phlegm. It worked.

As in this case, my father's successes often resulted from using fewer as opposed to more antibiotics, an approach he had learned early on from Louis Weinstein and one that he would impart to generations of Case Western Reserve medical students, house officers and fellows. One woman with multiple myeloma, who had been admitted repeatedly for infections, had a pneumonia that would not respond to any treatment. Given her overall condition, my dad, thinking it was cruel "to put her through any more torture," recommended that antibiotics be withdrawn and the patient made comfortable. The pneumonia, or whatever the lung condition was, resolved.

In another case, a woman had severe diarrhea probably related to previous use of an antimicrobial. A visiting professor had seen the patient and recommended "massive antibiotic therapy" to clear out what he thought was an infection in the intestines. But my father had noticed that in addition to the diarrhea, there was mucus in the stool, indicating that the patient's immune system was already fighting the diarrhea. He recommended stopping all antibiotics and simply giving her sugar water, "the way one would treat an infantile diarrhea." The patient recovered over the next several days.

Finally, my father consulted on a man who had been admitted with three weeks of high temperatures from an unclear source, a condition termed *fever of unexplained origin* (FUO) in a well-known 1961 paper by Paul Beeson and his Yale colleague Robert Petersdorf. With antibiotics, the patient's fevers had come down but had not gone away. My dad convinced his colleagues to avoid any further invasive testing and send the patient home. They agreed, and the temperatures gradually disappeared.

So how did my father instinctively know when to be aggressive and when to cut back? He would have cited his clinical expertise, beginning with his years as a medical resident and an infectious diseases fellow in Boston and continuing with his experience as an attending physician in Cleveland. Indeed, after the case described

above, he planned to compile a series of his FUO cases, those patients "who spontaneously recover without any definitive diagnosis
and without ever again getting into trouble." This, after all, was
the sort of clinical research that my father did during his years in
Cleveland—retrospective studies of cases that shared a common
characteristic, usually infections caused by a particular rare organism. The research was top-notch and published in excellent, peer-
reviewed journals. In order to improve his knowledge and conduct
his research, my dad diligently tracked down patients who had been
discharged, often sending them personal letters.

But my father's style of research belonged to an earlier era.
By the late 1970s, the randomized clinical trial—in which large
numbers of patients were enrolled in formal studies and followed
prospectively over time—had come into ascendancy. Researchers
sought major grants from the National Institutes of Health (NIH)
and often collaborated at multiple medical centers throughout the
country. Only through this type of sophisticated scientific analysis, biostatisticians argued, could true knowledge be obtained. Case
studies like those done by my father were interesting but not necessarily representative.

Still, on any given day at any given hospital, consultants like my
dad and Weinstein could amaze colleagues, students, and patients.
In one instance, the VA doctors asked my father to see an unusual
case of pneumonia that had stumped everyone. But he knew this
bacterium well. "It was *Nocardia*," Robert Bonomo, who trained
under my dad, told me a few years ago. "He came over and nailed
it." On another occasion, when several physicians were evaluating a
complicated skin infection, my dad was the only doctor present who
knew all the planes of tissue where bacteria could hide. J. Walton
Tomford, another Cleveland infectious diseases specialist, fondly
recalled attending the citywide conference at which my father and
the two other local infectious diseases gurus, Marty McHenry and
Manny Wolinsky, had the opportunity to show off their vast knowledge about the field—even taking one another on at times. "It was
like our church and synagogue," Tomford told me. These doctors
also loved to visit their colleagues' hospitals. In one memorable case,

my father asked McHenry to come to the Mount Sinai to convince a very reluctant Orthodox Jewish woman that she needed to have a lung biopsy. When McHenry, a devout Catholic, took out his rosary to pray for the woman, she quickly acquiesced.

In another instance, when no source of infection could be found in an older woman with a high fever, my father suggested that an artery along the side of her head—which was not at all tender—be biopsied to look for inflammation. The medical literature suggested that the condition he was looking for, temporal arteritis, caused only low-grade temperatures in the elderly, but my dad had seen three other cases with high fever. To the surprise of everyone, even my father, the biopsy was positive and the diagnosis was made. "This really represents the evolution of a consultant's experience," he subsequently wrote.

Once, an internist asked him to see a young woman who had developed a rash on her right forearm several days after receiving the antimicrobial ampicillin for a fever and sore throat. My father saw her at her home because she lived near us. I presume he took with him his black doctor's bag, which he used for his infrequent house calls and which contained the slides, syringes, and other equipment he needed to make a diagnosis. The rash was very distinctive, extending in a linear pattern from her elbow to her wrist. It was petechial—that is, composed of small purple spots caused by broken blood vessels. My dad immediately suspected meningococcemia, the severe bacterial blood infection on which his future mentor Weinstein had been lecturing on the day they met in 1960. Employing a bit of showmanship, my father asked the woman if she had recently been playing tennis. Startled, she said that she had, a few days before, around the time she had first seen her internist. He later attributed this feat of clinical acumen to the concept of *locus minoris resistentiae* (place of least resistance), taught to him by Weinstein. Due to the vigorous motion in the patient's forearm caused by playing tennis, the meningococcal bacteria had preferentially settled there and caused a rash. Before leaving, my dad put a drop of liquid from one of the lesions onto a slide, returned to the hospital, and did his own Gram stain, confirming the diagnosis.

In yet another case, my father overruled an "excellent internist and competent ophthalmologist" and prescribed a low dose of an antileukemia drug for a woman who had shingles that involved her eye. The patient's symptoms dramatically improved by the next morning. The basis of his decision? Observations that he and an infectious diseases colleague at nearby University Hospital had made that, in fact, contradicted a controlled study of the medication that had recently been done at the NIH. "Another aspect of the case that is certainly worth commenting on is the beautiful demonstration of the value of a specialist in a given situation," my dad later wrote. "This is really a minutia type of therapeutic maneuver and can only come about through word of mouth and personal experience." Although he closely reviewed the results of major clinical trials, he passionately asserted that keen clinical observation remained the most important way to approach illness and care for sick people.

To what degree was my father truly bucking the trend in medicine that increasingly favored population-based data over clinical intuition? In her 2013 book on Sister Kenny, the famous polio nurse of the 1930s and 1940s, the historian Naomi Rogers argues that Kenny actually constructed an alternative pathophysiological model of the disease based on her personal bedside observations. That is, she rejected the then-current scientific explanations for how polio crippled patients, feeling that the mechanism responsible was the muscle spasms she observed, as opposed to nerve damage. Kenny's novel treatment strategy for polio, which involved mobilizing paralyzed muscles as early as possible, followed directly from her unorthodox perspective. Seeing, in other words, was believing. I encountered this epistemological conundrum when researching breast cancer: certain patients insisted that their cancers were caused by toxic exposures and others assured me that screening mammograms had saved their lives even though controlled-study data indicated that both scenarios were unlikely.

Firmly grounded in scientific medicine, my father did not hold radical beliefs. But he practiced what the sociologist Charles L. Bosk called, in his 1979 book on surgical training, "clinical individualism." My dad believed that his observations and research constituted a type of clinical reality that was lost when physicians considered only the characteristics of a given disease among large populations of patients. More provocatively, he thought that doctors could use their clinical acumen, experience, and even empathy to reach conclusions about how specific illnesses acted or were likely to act in specific patients. Without scientific proof, of course, these claims could always be contested. But for my father and those trained in a similar manner, such insights needed to be considered at patients' bedsides.

Regardless of their beliefs about how medical knowledge was best generated, my dad's colleagues largely appreciated his insights and were glad to have a meticulous, experienced, and compassionate physician looking over their shoulders. But he was not universally beloved. My father had extremely high standards and little tolerance for those who he believed were lazy or incompetent. If a patient needed antibiotics emergently and was not getting them, according to Robert Bonomo, my dad would yell, "You need to do this now!" until it happened. In one instance, my father learned that a senior surgeon was planning to follow his usual routine and give a penicillin compound to a patient who was already on the operating table. Believing that the patient had a penicillin allergy, my father went to the operating room and demanded that the patient be given a different antibiotic. The situation was tense but Phil Lerner ultimately prevailed. In his early years as a consultant, my father weighed carefully "the pros and cons of stepping on toes." Later in his career, he often directly confronted certain colleagues, which probably contributed to an informal nickname that he acquired over the years: the Madman of the Mount Sinai.

My father justified such conduct by an intense devotion to his patients, which emanated from his upbringing and training and was, for him, the heart of medical practice. He went the extra mile not only to comfort his patients but also to demonstrate behaviors that he hoped other doctors might emulate. Of course, my dad's ability to sit down with patients, spend time with them, and answer their questions was enhanced by his job as a consultant in the postwar, pre–managed-care era. Paul Beeson had advocated the same humanistic approach. So did fictional television doctor Marcus Welby, who was on the air from 1969 to 1976.

A representative case was that of a twenty-eight-year-old woman admitted for severe intestinal bleeding and several related complications whom my father described as "emotionally-shocked," "terribly sick," and "frightened." Even though she turned out not to have an infection, my dad was the one who calmed her down during a "fantastic screaming spell" that he suspected was due to the "frightening stillness" of the regular ward once she had left the "hustle and bustle" of intensive care. Appreciating his kindness, the woman relied on him both during and after her hospital stay. "A very rewarding experience," he later wrote, "but really outside my primary area of interest." So, too, perhaps, was the time that he spent a half hour speaking with a woman with a severe bone infection who had become upset when one of her other physicians had made a light-hearted remark about her condition. Another patient my father bonded intensely with was a young man who showed "considerable fortitude and maturity" while battling ultimately incurable endocarditis. Although my dad strove to maintain a strictly "professional relationship" with his patients, he admitted that he had developed a "genuine affection" for this man.

One of my father's more interesting encounters involved a patient who wrote to him to protest what he believed was an excessive fee for a ten-minute consultation. My dad wrote him back and explained that the consult had also involved discussions with the man's doctors and nurses as well as a review of his chart and X-rays. The patient was evidently impressed because he paid the entire bill and added in an extra five dollars for the time it had taken my father to write a reply. This gesture was perhaps the 1970s equivalent of paying the doctor with a chicken. The five dollars was, of course, returned. This encounter was quintessential Phil Lerner: he went the extra mile to explain and demonstrate his philosophy of doctoring, and he gained a patient and a friend in the process.

My father was hardly the only intensely engaged physician at the Mount Sinai. Much more so than today's practitioners, doctors of my dad's generation viewed the medical decisions they made as almost personal—and defended them with ardor. My father was even known to get into fights with his brother, Allan, himself a passionate patient advocate. Once, when my dad noticed a house officer watching him and his brother argue with each other about a particular case, my father turned to the resident, rolled his eyes, and asked, "See what I have to put up with?" On another occasion, my father walked into the medical intensive care unit to find a surgeon and a gastroenterologist who disagreed about a patient's care actually *physically* fighting with each other. In this case, my dad served as a peacemaker, helping to pull the two men apart. Recalling what he regarded as the Mount Sinai's heyday, he later wrote that he "could bring any of my patients or anyone of my family into this hospital with the absolute assurance that the finest medical care was available in a stimulating, friendly and warm environment where everyone took pride in their work and was rewarded with the satisfaction of a job well done, even when the patient ran into problems, and even when death was the final chapter."

My father's concern for his patients was only enhanced by the fact that so many of them had a personal connection to him. Having lived most of his life in Cleveland and its suburbs, he knew many Jewish families. Of course, he also had personal connections to many non-Jewish patients, who were often former classmates, friends, and colleagues. In the words of the historian David J. Rothman, "doctor and patient occupied the same social space," promoting a shared relationship. Meanwhile, the poor and minority patients my dad met for the first time at the Mount Sinai—including many he would then follow for years—got the same royal treatment. Just as my father's choice of profession was in part out of gratitude that he'd grown up an ocean away from the Holocaust, his devotion to these ward or service patients, as they were called, was his way of acknowledging his good luck in the face of so many ongoing catastrophes around the globe. His goal was to "take extra pains with the service patients, to be certain they are reassured and confident in your care, and come to believe that you really care about him or her as an individual." One way he did this was to take advantage of his flexible schedule. "It's so simple," he wrote, "to make an extra visit in the afternoon for these special cases, come back to report a new lab test result, review an X-ray [or] reassure that the scheduled test is necessary, important and will lead to some conclusive information." Illness, he underscored, was "frightening." When I read these words many years later as a professor, I had to smile. It was the exact sort of advice that I gave to students and residents when teaching them about the history of medicine and the doctor-patient relationship. My dad had acted this way as a matter of course.

Another group of my father's patients consisted of doctors, nurses, other hospital employees, and their relatives. There may be no higher compliment for a physician than to be asked to care for a colleague's loved ones, and my dad was definitely a "doctor's doctor." The 1970s was still an era of professional courtesy, and my father generally waived or reduced his fees when treating coworkers or their family members. This concept of the medical profession as a sort of guild that looked out for its members was a comforting one and may even have contributed to my decision to become a doctor. I remember seeing a few of my dad's peers for sundry medical issues and feeling as if I was in good hands.

Whether he was caring for a friend, a relative, or a stranger, my father's clinical interactions were always dominated by a paternalistic philosophy. It made sense to him that, since physicians trained for decades, spent long hours in the hospital, and devoted themselves to the care of both the poor and the wealthy, they should call the shots, and patients should acquiesce. Doctor knew best, whether he—and it was usually a he in those days—was renowned Harvard surgeon Francis Moore, polio vaccine inventor Jonas Salk, or heart transplant pioneer Christiaan Barnard. Practicing any other way was an abrogation of one's duty. Physicians of my father's era saw their paternalism as not only altruistic, but therapeutic: it was widely believed that if patients followed doctors' *orders* (and that is what therapies and other interventions were called), they were more likely to recover. Sometimes in serious illness, New York infectious diseases specialist Walsh McDermott said, the physician himself was the treatment.

Perhaps the best example of how paternalism dominated medicine was the fact that physicians in the postwar era routinely lied to cancer patients about their diagnoses. Doctors jumped through all sorts of hoops to try to convince their patients—many of whom were dying of their disease—that they had merely a tumor or an inflammation. Surgery and radiation therapy, the patients were told, were given "to be on the safe side." When Columbia nephrologist Jay I. Meltzer joined a group practice of more senior physicians, he soon realized that "the best doctors were," paradoxically, "the best liars." He demurred, preferring to find out from patients in advance what they would or would not like to know about their diagnoses. Meltzer told me a story about paternalism involving his former Columbia colleague and devoted physician Randolph Bailey. After learning of the famous 1964 surgeon general's report delineating the dangers of cigarettes, Bailey had told Meltzer that he planned to keep smoking so that his patients, who were unlikely to be able to stop themselves anyway, would not feel "frightened and helpless."

Thanks to the large number of clinical advances in the postwar years—many of which came from experimental research—the medical profession at this time was gaining enormous prestige. The new antimicrobial agents had made formerly ubiquitous and scary diseases, like syphilis, tuberculosis, and bacterial pneumonia, far more manageable. The discovery and synthesis of insulin meant diabetes was very treatable. Salk's vaccine had led to dramatically lower rates of polio, the dreaded summer plague. Meanwhile, the ability to bank blood made possible more aggressive operations for aneurysms, cancer, and other conditions. By the early 1960s, there were medications to treat high blood pressure, and dialysis machines to prolong the lives of patients with severe kidney disease. It was no longer enough to simply be a kindly and caring physician; the public also wanted doctors who were engaged with the latest laboratory research. "If They Can Operate, You're Lucky" was the tagline for a cover story in the May 3, 1963, edition of *Time* magazine that detailed several innovative and aggressive new operations.

From a modern vantage point, it may seem curious that patients were so passive when dealing with such a serious topic as life-threatening illness. And there have always been patients who have questioned their doctors and disregarded their advice. But many sick people welcomed the opportunity to have highly trained profession-als make all their decisions. One explanatory model for this behav-ior, introduced by Harvard University sociologist Talcott Parsons in 1951, was called the sick role. Relieved of their normal duties due to their illnesses, patients believed they had an obligation to do what was necessary to get well, specifically by cooperating in the therapeutic process. Thus, while Columbia professor Robert Loeb's domineering personality bothered some patients, most revered him. After all, the man was in the hospital seven days a week and knew the names of all his patients, their family members, and even the hospital janitors. The same admiration was shown to breast surgeon Jerome Urban, who pioneered the super-radical mastectomy, a dra-matic operation in which a woman's breastbone and ribs were re-moved in an attempt to get rid of elusive cancer cells. Urban often slept on the couch in his office so he would be available to resume operating first thing in the morning. Long after such disfiguring surgery had been discredited, Urban's patients remained quite cer-tain his extraordinary efforts had saved their lives. Late at night, Columbia-Presbyterian surgeon Philip Wiedel pushed a small cart down the hospital's corridor, quietly entering patients' rooms and changing their dressings by himself. "A doctor must work 18 hours a day and seven days a week," wrote one physician from this era. "If you cannot console yourself to this, get out of the profession."

But by the early 1970s, the situation had begun to change. Over the previous decade, a series of research scandals revealed that some physicians had been willing to put fame and science above their con-cerns for patients. These violations occurred despite the fact that the Nuremberg Code—written in 1946 in response to the inhumane experiments carried out by Nazi physicians during the Holocaust—had explicitly mandated that all subjects must give informed consent before being enrolled in research. Yet in one case, a doctor studying the body's immune response to cancer had actually injected cancer cells into the skin of chronically ill noncancer patients at a hospital in Brooklyn. These individuals, many of whom were, ironically, Ho-locaust survivors, were told only that they needed an injection. And what about the deliberate administration of active hepatitis virus into physically and mentally disabled children at the Willowbrook State School on Staten Island? The researchers argued that since there were frequent outbreaks of hepatitis at the institution, these children would get the disease anyway, and the study might lead to a preventive vaccine. But wasn't this doing harm to a population that could not consent? The outrage reached a peak in 1972 when an Associated Press reporter revealed that in Tuskegee, Alabama, the US Public Health Service had observed poor southern African American men with syphilis for as long as forty years in order to study the "natural history" of the disease. The researchers had even continued the experiment—depriving the men of treatment—when a highly curative antibiotic, penicillin, became available in the 1940s. Many of the subjects died of syphilis as a result of this deception. That the men in the Tuskegee study were black and the doctors who conducted research at major medical centers were overwhelmingly white was especially objectionable in an era of civil rights protests.

Meanwhile, some women with breast cancer were in almost full-fledged revolt. For decades, surgeons had done biopsies of breast lumps while women were under anesthesia. If the biopsies were positive, the surgeons believed immediate radical mastectomies were indicated. Rather than awakening their patients to obtain consent, they preferred to forge ahead with the procedure, although if a woman was married, the surgeon would ask the husband's permission. When a woman awoke from this operation, she commonly reached for her chest to see whether or not her breast was still there, an experience that many described as thoroughly traumatic. In the early 1970s, with the support of an iconoclastic surgeon from the Cleveland Clinic, George Crile Jr., a group of activist women began to refuse both this combination procedure and the reflexive use of such a mutilating radical operation for small, localized breast cancers. The best known of these women was Rose Kushner, a Washington, DC, journalist whose story I was privileged to tell in *The Breast Cancer Wars*, my book on the history of breast cancer. Confronted by this feminist initiative, most breast surgeons initially became more—not less—paternalistic, and at times patronizing. For example, in 1971, another journalist, Babette Rosmond, got her surgeon to agree to do just the biopsy of a breast lump. But when it came back positive and she asked for a few weeks to consider her options rather than immediately undergoing a radical mastectomy, he called her "a silly and stubborn woman" and made the ridiculous claim that she might be dead in a few weeks without the procedure.

By the mid-1970s, historians and other authors began to portray the medical profession and the history of medicine in an unflattering light. *Medical Nemesis,* by the Austrian philosopher Ivan Illich, argued that doctors did far more harm than good. Patients, he wrote, were "defenseless" against "the damage that doctors inflict with the intent of curing." In *The Birth of the Clinic,* French historian Michel Foucault saw paternalism as a cloak that gave physicians far too much power and, paradoxically, also distanced them from patients.

Neither a breast surgeon nor a gynecologist, my father was less likely to encounter these new activist patients. But issues of patients' rights were slowly creeping into his world, and at times, his notes contained a glimmer of the coming revolution. For example, one of his patients developed congestive heart failure due to endocarditis but, against the advice of my dad and a cardiologist, was able to successfully maintain a very vigorous exercise program. "We have a situation," my father wrote, "where the patient, either out of ignorance, or fear, teaches the consultant something and challenges some traditional concepts." Cases like this reminded my dad that even when he relied on his best medical judgment, he was not necessarily right.

More interesting was a case in which an orthopedic surgeon disregarded my father's advice regarding an infected elbow without telling the patient what had been recommended. My dad, in contrast to the surgeon, thought that the elbow needed to be opened up and drained. My father later wrote that he did not know where his "legal, moral and ethical duty would reside" in this circumstance, but that "ideally," he would "ignore the surgeon and directly tell the patient what I believe that the proper treatment should be and recommend that she seek this from some other source." In this instance, at least, the etiquette of not stepping on his colleague's toes won out over the patient's right to know my dad's contrary opinion.

He did not go behind the orthopedist's back and talk to the patient. But the decision clearly made him uncomfortable.

Coincidentally, twenty years later, when running a session on bioethical dilemmas, I heard a very similar case, one in which a neurosurgeon was insisting on inserting a drain into the head of a boy despite the fact that the radiologist had told the house staff that it was not needed. When asked whether I thought the younger doctors had an ethical obligation to go over the senior surgeon's head and inform the boy's parents about this disagreement, my answer was an unequivocal yes. In an era of patient autonomy, they simply had the right to know. One can sense my father struggling here to incorporate new ethical norms into a very powerful and familiar style of medicine that he had long believed was best. It was a difficult task.

The tension between doctors' prerogatives and patients' rights came to a head, most commonly, in questions of medical error. Traditionally, hospitals had dealt with these problems internally, either informally among the involved physicians or at morbidity and mortality conferences. Although mistakes might be admitted during such reviews with the goal of making sure they did not happen again, any acknowledgments of guilt were kept secret from patients, families, and even uninvolved coworkers. The fear of lawsuits was simply too overwhelming. Thus, my father often used errors he had witnessed to provide himself and his colleagues with important lessons for the future, such as "It's not necessarily gangrene just because there is some gas in the tissues" and "You can't use a reduced dosage of Loridine in patients who have renal dysfunction." What to do about the problem of medical errors more broadly was not addressed. In one particularly disturbing case, the father of a young man with a possible brain abscess kept interfering with the efforts of my dad and the other doctors to obtain a diagnostic arteriogram because the test was invasive and involved the injection of dye. As the negotiations persisted, the patient suddenly became comatose: he did have an abscess and it had ruptured, a true medical emergency that might have been avoided. Fortunately, the man survived. Not doing what was best for his patient, my father concluded, had been a huge mistake. "It will never happen again as far as I'm concerned," he wrote. But, as usual, no larger investigation into the case by the hospital hierarchy ensued.

My father's reticence to go public extended to cases in which patients had been mismanaged prior to being admitted to the hospital. Some patients' serious illnesses could be traced to questionable diagnostic or therapeutic choices made by previous clinicians. In one case, for example, my dad saw a woman for pneumonia and realized that none of the other doctors had found her very obviously enlarged neck lymph nodes, which indicated that the patient almost surely also had lung cancer. He likely never revealed that mistake to the patient. When a newborn baby developed a serious infection known as toxoplasmosis and my father was called in on the case very late, he experienced "true frustration." Although he was "not certain that earlier treatment would have made a difference," he believed that effective therapy had been available, "and it might have made the difference between a child totally retarded and institutionalized and perhaps a child who could have lived a more normal existence." Again, there is no suggestion in his journals that he ever said anything to the baby's parents. My father thought that he could be a more effective consultant by educating his colleagues about their errors and reminding them when and why they should call him. But that is where it ended, at least well into the 1980s. A consultant, he wrote, had to be "extremely careful in what he says" to patients and families. Under the ethical codes of the era, the sanctity of the doctor-doctor relationship still took precedence.

But my father remained conflicted about this sort of silence and made some gestures that—if not open admissions of errors—acknowledged bad outcomes. In one case, a teenage boy had died of an extremely severe pneumonia that his pediatrician had not originally taken seriously. My dad, who described himself as "shaken by this case," asked the referring physician if he might seek out the family and explain what had taken place. "I did this," my father wrote, "and it was not a very pleasant task." I suspect that, in addition to expressing his condolences, my dad focused on the medical aspects of the case. In another instance, he typed up a three-page single-spaced note for his own files about a boy who had died of severe liver disease after bouncing in and out of several hospitals. "Given the final diagnosis and a treatable disease, could we have expected to save this youngster?" he asked himself. "I think the answer is yes and no." My father attended the several-hour autopsy but called the "cold and austere" autopsy room "chilling" and felt that he was the only person in attendance with any emotional connection to the case. There is no mention of a postmortem visit with the parents in this instance, but it was this type of complicated case that bioethicists would soon urge physicians to openly discuss with patients and their families.

Being a full-time academic meant that in addition to seeing infectious diseases consults at the Mount Sinai and neighboring hospitals, my father taught medical students and house officers and sat on various medical school and hospital administrative committees. He also regularly read up to twelve medical journals, both those devoted to his specialty and others meant for the larger medical community. Keeping up with the literature was essential for any practicing clinician, but particularly for the consultant, who was relied upon for the latest knowledge about new medications and recent scientific studies. Not knowing all such information would have been an abrogation of one's duty. As was the case in the homes of many doctors of this era, our bookshelves were lined with volumes of certain medical journals that my dad had read and, at the end of each year, had bound. This information was also available at the medical school, but having a home library ever available for consultation was important. In the days before the Internet simplified researching the scientific literature, my father would rip out articles on interesting cases from various journals. When encountering a similar case at work, a lightbulb would go on and he would try to find the jagged pages he had stuck, most often, in a poorly labeled folder. At one point he wrote that some people were "incredulous" that he had no interest in golf, bridge, or other hobbies, but he nonetheless remained focused on increasing his medical knowledge, studying his profession.

My dad's passion for medical research came through vividly in an anecdote I found in his journals about a national infectious diseases conference that he attended. A speaker there had presented exciting data on a new modality, monoclonal antibodies, that held enormous potential for the treatment of infections and cancers. Someone in the audience asked why he had not mentioned the earlier work of another researcher, leading the speaker to praise that investigator's work, which had gone largely unappreciated. Then another hand went up in the audience. It was the earlier researcher himself, who then recounted his saga, adding that the Nobel Prize–winning immunologist Macfarlane Burnet had once come up to him on a London bus to commend him for "immortalizing the cell that makes antibody."

"The audience went wild," my father wrote, "well, at least as wild as that type of audience could muster."

It is not hard to understand why he included this event in his journals. Monoclonal antibodies were the exact type of scientific breakthrough that had drawn my father to infectious diseases in the late 1950s, as the nascent specialty was conquering tuberculosis, polio, and other dread diseases. There was nothing quite so exciting in medicine as learning about a new technology that might save the lives of otherwise doomed patients.

My dad fanatically followed his own patients, even when we were on vacation. He scheduled daily calls from Cape Cod or wherever we were staying to review the cases with the residents or fellows covering the infectious diseases service. We traveled only at the end of the month so that the covering doctors would know the service well, a habit that struck me as utterly inconceivable once my wife and I began the arduous task of planning family vacations that suited all our schedules. In later years, when my parents vacationed each June with my uncle in the south of France, my father still kept tabs on his patients. A June 1990 journal entry noted that he was "consumed with worrying about my patients" and had dreamed about the sickest one the previous night. I am not positive, but I suspect he himself paid for the phone calls from France to Cleveland. Indeed, as the only infectious diseases specialist at Mount Sinai, he was technically on call every day he worked there from 1973 until 1993, when he finally hired an associate. And yet, as Robert Bonomo reminded

me, my omnipresent father always made sure to let his younger colleagues "spread their wings." "What are you trying to achieve?" was
one of his favorite questions to his trainees.

My father's various commitments left little time for the other
portion of his job: clinical research. The only time he could do
this activity was on nights and weekends. And that's when he did
it. Pretty much every night after dinner, if he was not attending
a meeting, he would spend hours reading and writing at a table
crowded with books and journals. Within the house, my dad was
sort of a wandering Jew. For a while, he used the kitchen table after
it had been cleared. However, this necessitated reorganizing and removing the materials every night before he went to bed. So at some
point, he commandeered the less-used dining-room table, which
could serve as a more permanent repository. The fourth bedroom
upstairs, his home office, was piled high with journals, books, and
medical charts. New York City gastroenterologist and author Michael Lepore called the colleagues of his who spent their free time
doing extra patient care, teaching, and researching the "sons of Hippocrates," physicians who "gave more than they took." My dad was
doing the same thing five hundred miles to the west.

I grew up thinking that my father's constant work was essential
and commonplace. With important knowledge to soak up and papers to write, he did what he had to do. Sure, it made him less available to his family, but my admiration for his diligence substantially
outweighed whatever frustration I felt. Once I was a teenager, I was
just as glad to have him occupied and not bothering me. My sister, however, later admitted that she had felt that his work habits
were excessive and even selfish. For my mother, her spouse's constant immersion in medicine was one of many sacrifices she had had
to make in marrying a physician who was both an academic and a
workaholic. Having now read his journals, I see that publishing his
findings was his way of keeping alive the sort of case-based clinical
knowledge that he believed was disappearing.

Meanwhile, I was growing up, staying at Hawken School for both
middle and upper school. Decades later, when I began researching
events in the history of medicine in the 1960s and 1970s, I was glad

that I had started Hawken in 1969. The formal traditions that I experienced at the school must have provided a reassuring contrast with the social turmoil that had come to Cleveland, mostly in the form of riots in the largely African American Hough area that abutted Case Western Reserve and its affiliated hospitals. On at least one occasion, the police prevented my father from getting to the Veterans Administration hospital due to violence in the area. Hawken stayed immune for as long as it could. When I started there as a fourth grader in 1969, we called all the male teachers "sir" and stood whenever a female entered the room. Before winter and summer vacations, each student formally shook hands with the entire faculty. Within a couple of years, all these customs, plus the dress code, seemed antiquated and had been relaxed. But my Hawken experiences reminded me about the varying ways in which social change spreads in different communities.

A notable event during my middle school years was my bar mitzvah. There had been no question that my father would have an Orthodox bar mitzvah, given his religious household. But, in part due to his subsequent ambivalence about Judaism, our family had never even joined a temple. By the time I got around to deciding to forge ahead, at age twelve, the only Hebrew school willing to prepare me for the event was a local Orthodox school, Yeshiva Adath B'nai Israel, located about a mile from my house. The fact that I was the son of a noted Cleveland doctor probably did not hurt in their decision to accept me as a student. Not surprisingly, YABI was like a different world for me, although one my Eastern European ancestors would have recognized. The male teachers dressed in black, had long beards, and wore traditional yarmulkes and tzitzit. The women were second-class citizens and, to my chagrin, had to sit separately from the men at services. Like my father, I had little use for the prayers.

Ultimately, however, I was glad I had a bar mitzvah. All four of my grandparents, plus my great-grandfather Ben, attended. My grandfather Meyer, upset that my father had largely renounced his faith, was thrilled that the service was Orthodox, allowing me to chant in Hebrew for close to two hours. It was especially meaningful to me that Ben, by then a widower and in his eighties, was there. Here was a man who had left Poland without his family or money, somehow leapfrogging over the Holocaust, and who was now attending his great-grandson's Orthodox bar mitzvah in America. I hope my performance that day was at least partial payback for the remarkable path my ancestors had followed.

And my experiences at YABI were a good stepping-stone for my future career studying bioethics and history. The biblical stories we discussed in class, populated with just and heroic characters (usually Jews) and readily identifiable villains (occasionally Jews, but usually not), were full of ethical lessons about right and wrong. And I recall some provocative discussions about whether these stories were historically accurate or merely moralistic tales that anonymous scholars had penned. I also enjoyed questioning the seemingly straightforward religious traditions that Rabbi Joseph Fabian and the teachers passed down to the school's students. For example, I remember asking why YABI members offered to come into our homes with some type of blowtorch to remove every last bit of bread (*chametz* in Hebrew) in our cabinets in preparation for the Passover holidays. "Isn't the symbolic act of eating no bread for eight days much more important than whether or not you accidentally leave a few crumbs lying around?" I asked. The teacher, as I recall, was appalled at my heresy. The medical profession, I would later learn, could be just as dogmatic about its traditions and beliefs.

Meanwhile, middle school was a challenge. I had gained weight, developed a bad case of acne, and, perhaps worst of all, become very socially awkward. As Hawken was still an all-boys school, I had fewer and fewer interactions with girls. My major outside interest was sports.

Plus, I was in conflict with my father. "Barron, I don't know at all," he wrote in 1977. "He's a closed creature, a self-contained enigma." In my defense, this characterization probably applies to a lot of teenagers. And the apple did not fall far from the tree. My dad kept his emotions locked away as well. The thing that bothered him most was my academic performance—or lack of it. Accustomed to my getting all As, he did not understand why this was no longer the case and why it did not bother me more. Truth be told, I don't really know the answer myself. One's teenage years are generally a time of rebellion, but, aside from my solitary nature, I was essentially a Boy Scout. I had no allowance and earned my spending money with a paper route that required me to get up at six in the morning. Moreover, there were neither girls nor drugs nor secret parties; I did not even talk back to my parents. Once I was eighteen, I drank only on weekends and moderately. In fact, after I got my driver's license, I became the de facto designated driver for my friends, even before the concept had gained currency in this country. My friends and I were fairly quintessential nerds, bonding over sports and ogling girls, undoubtedly to their dismay.

So perhaps taking it easy at school was my brand of revolt. In retrospect, I was probably exhausted. I remember staying up most nights to watch the monologue on Johnny Carson's *Tonight* show, which meant that I was getting only six hours of sleep much of the time. And I was not doing terribly, by any means, just Bs along with my As. I think most of my father's frustration stemmed from his own childhood history. Having had a father who had been forced to drop out of school, he had busted his butt at academics while also working part-time jobs. But here I was, attending a prestigious private school and seemingly not doing my best. When I got what he believed were bad report cards, he would yell at me and then give me the silent treatment. Typical of the era's wives and mothers, my mom quietly tried to defend me but never really challenged my father's authority.

Some subjects certainly interested me more than others. My first love was history. Going back to my early obsession with the presidents, I had always been fascinated with the past and would read for hours about old sports events, movies, buildings, and political figures. Many of my sixth-grade classmates were bored during a trip to the Henry Ford Museum and Dearborn Village, but I remember staring intently at the early-twentieth-century cars and gasoline pumps, even imagining myself living in that era. I was very nostalgic as a kid and have remained so as an adult. History tests were always easy for me, as I was a great memorizer of facts and an above-average writer. As a high school senior, I became the coeditor of the peculiarly named school newspaper, the *Affirmative No.* I also did fine in math, biology, chemistry, and physics, which would help me as a premed in college.

My summers were largely spent at home, aside from the annual late August vacation to beautiful Wellfleet on Cape Cod. I bypassed the opportunity to go to sleepaway camp. A typical summer for me was spent doing my paper route and either going to a local day camp or taking classes at the public high school. I also "worked" for my father, requesting reprints for him of medical articles—often from obscure journals—the titles of which he had found interesting. In an era before the Internet and Medline, exchanging reprints was an important way for physicians to share information. I also sent out reprints of my dad's articles. Even though many requests for them came from South America, Europe, and Asia, and thus required extra postage, my father saw the opportunity to share his work as an honor. My job, for which I was reimbursed, was tedious, but once again I admired my dad's zeal for obtaining and disseminating medical knowledge.

In the summer of 1975, between ninth and tenth grades, I embarked on a new activity. In addition to his other tasks, my father had become the medical director of Montefiore, a nursing home started under Jewish auspices and located in Cleveland Heights, about a twenty-minute bicycle ride from my house. Most of the medical problems among the residents were not infectious in nature, but my father was also a highly competent internist. I suspect he took the job mostly for the extra paycheck it brought in.

As with other nursing homes, Montefiore encouraged teenagers to volunteer as "friendly visitors." In taking on this position, my main task was to keep the residents company, either in their rooms, outside, or in the small coffee shop. Why did my father want me to volunteer at Montefiore? Perhaps, as with the not-too-subtle interesting clinical vignettes he frequently told me, it was part of his plan to push me toward a career in medicine. But I suspect that it was more related to his larger campaign to get me interested in something other than sports. As usual, I complied with his suggestion. The fact that two cute girls from the public high school were also volunteering there probably did more to motivate me than anything else.

But once I started working there, I had to admit that I liked it. One of my earliest memories is my father taking me upstairs to the nursing home's second floor, which was essentially a large dayroom for patients who needed full-time supervision. He introduced me to an elderly man, impeccably dressed in a suit and tie, who had been the chairman of medicine at one of the local hospitals. We chatted briefly and he wished me luck. When my father and I went back downstairs, I asked him what such an impressive individual was doing in that location. "He is completely demented," I was told. "He no longer has any idea of where he is." It was my first encounter with Alzheimer's disease and an utterly vivid demonstration of how a healthy body could house a severely dysfunctional brain.

I still remember the first two residents I visited. One, named Esther, was a warm and very talkative woman who probably qualified as the nursing-home gossip. The second, Max, was a polite and generous man who reminded me of my grandfather Meyer. Truth be told, neither of these people needed a volunteer. They were among the most high-functioning and sociable residents of the home. But I assumed that the head of volunteers liked to start out her new charges with simple cases. I eased into my position as a volunteer with little difficulty. I had always been a child who was quite comfortable speaking with adults; I showed them respect, used humor when appropriate, and was eager to hear their stories. Later on, my older patients would often tell me I was the only doctor who listened to them, surely an exaggeration but something I was nevertheless pleased to hear.

The most memorable resident of Montefiore at the time was someone we would now call high maintenance. Ed was wheelchair-bound, for reasons I could never quite understand, and highly emotional. He used his feet to move his wheelchair around the premises, constantly getting into other people's business. When he learned that I was Phil Lerner's son, he started crying, an event that would repeat itself many times. He would then proceed to rave about how my father was the most wonderful doctor he had ever met and how I was so lucky to have him as a father.

Such unbridled emotion made me uncomfortable, especially if either of the two girls I liked was around. But I could not help but be moved. My dad did something for a living that really made a difference to people. Even though I probably hated him at the time for putting so much pressure on me, I could see what his intense devotion achieved for people in need of not only medical care but an interested friend. When I read his journals thirty-five years later, I came to understand how the combination of scientific knowledge, clinical judgment, and prolonged face-to-face contact with patients and families enabled a physician to truly excel at his or her craft.

It was my experience at Montefiore that led me to seriously consider becoming a doctor. "I'm delighted," my father wrote to me on my fifteenth birthday, "that you show this evidence of empathy and willingness to help those less fortunate than yourself." I returned to the nursing home for a second summer in 1976. I still had no dates, however, with either the Montefiore girls or any others.

The next year, 1977, would be a devastating one for our family. My grandfather Meyer unexpectedly died, and my mother was diagnosed with breast cancer. We all took these events hard, but no one took them harder than my father. His relationship to medicine would never be the same.

CHAPTER THREE

Illness Hits Home

I still remember what my grandfather Meyer's legs looked like. They were pale and almost hairless, in direct contrast to the very hirsute ones shared by my father, me, and my son, Ben. They also had a large number of varicosities, collections of veins pushing up against the skin. Although they bothered him, the varicosities did not necessarily indicate major problems with the other blood vessels in his legs.

But those other veins are what most likely killed him. Recuperating in the hospital after routine surgery for a hernia, Meyer probably developed an undetected blood clot in his leg. At five in the morning on Easter Sunday, April 10, 1977, when he got up to go to the bathroom, it dislodged, traveled to his lung, and caused a fatal pulmonary embolism. That my father—his son the doctor—was in Iran made everything even worse.

We were still reeling from this tragedy when, two months later, my mother found a lump in her left breast. The biopsy showed cancer—which had spread to the lymph nodes. By the summer, she had undergone a mastectomy and was getting chemotherapy and experimental immunotherapy as part of a clinical trial. It was far from clear that she would survive.

That year, 1977, was a very bad year. The fact that both of these terrible events were health-related also had substantial ramifications. My father, accustomed to being in control of all things medical, now saw medicine as something that was causing powerlessness and pain. A sense of disenchantment with his career, which would accelerate over the coming years, began to creep into his journal entries. But at the same time, my grandfather's death and my mother's illness would contribute to my decision to commit to medicine.

Meyer was actually the third of the five grandparents who had been present at my 1973 bar mitzvah to die. Ben, Meyer's father, went first, in July 1974 at the age of eighty-six. Fittingly, given the role that religion had played in his move to America and the raising of his family, Ben died, presumably of a heart attack, at the local Jewish community center where he spent a few days a week "flirting with the old ladies."

Although I would eventually be a historian, I was not one yet. I don't recall ever asking Ben for tales of his life in Poland or while struggling to make a living in America. Writing this book, I have realized what a pity that is.

Mannie, my mother's father, was the next to die, in 1975. He and Jessie, who we called Poppa and Nana, had moved from Framingham in 1972 and joined us in University Heights. Soon after their arrival in Cleveland, Mannie began experiencing memory problems. The cause was probably a series of small strokes, as opposed to Alzheimer's, but after a while, he could no longer go unaccompanied to the nearby Cedar Center shopping area. His confusion gradually worsened. The cause of Mannie's death was never officially determined but it was likely due to a piece of intestine that had died, leading to septic shock and then the failure of the kidneys and other organs. It was the first family death that I would observe my father manage. At the age of fourteen, I assumed his therapeutic choices for his father-in-law had been entirely straightforward, but after I became a doctor, I realized that the situation had been more complicated. More family illnesses and deaths were on the way, including those of two of my grandmother Pearl's sisters. There was actually such a spate of deaths during the late 1970s that my sister thought that a man who was present at all the services—the director of the local Jewish funeral home—was our cousin.

But Meyer's death was by far the most jarring, and not only because he was still in his sixties. When we moved to Cleveland in 1966, we had actually lived with Meyer and Pearl for a few months while our new house was being readied. And during the next eleven years, we saw them often. Pearl was sharp-tongued, forever arguing with her sisters and fond of Yiddish slang. Meyer, by contrast, was a calm and gentle presence. He wore a shirt and tie at all times and a fedora hat when he went outside.

Despite their devotion to Judaism, Meyer and Pearl had never been to Israel. Part of the reason may have been the expense. While my father and his brother would gladly have helped them pay for it, their Depression mentality caused lifelong frugality. Of Pearl, my father wrote, "It's alien to her nature not to worry about money, and she'll never change." There were also, of course, safety concerns, especially prior to the 1978 Camp David treaty between Israel and Egypt.

My father had not been to Israel either. So when he was invited to be a visiting professor in, of all places, Shiraz, Iran, he decided to begin his trip with a week in the Jewish homeland. And, in an inspired move, he asked me to come. The first two weeks of his trip corresponded with my two-week spring vacation in eleventh grade, in March and April of 1977. The plan was that I would go with him, then fly home from Iran by myself, returning through Israel.

The trip was remarkable for a number of reasons. For one thing, it was an intense father-son bonding experience. My father was still displeased with my academic performance, but the trip was all about exploring our cultural heritage and seeing exciting tourist destinations. We rented a car in Israel and split most of our time between Tel Aviv and Jerusalem, with day trips to places like the Dead Sea and Masada. Particularly powerful was a visit to Kibbutz Dafna, near the southern border of Lebanon, where we stayed with relatives who had moved to Palestine before World War II.

And, of course, there was Yad Vashem, Israel's memorial to the victims of the Holocaust. My outwardly unemotional father was, I found out later, profoundly moved and disturbed. After I read his journals, I understood how this experience rekindled the feelings of guilt and the sense of good luck that had crafted his personality and helped guide his career in medicine. "The pictures at Yad Vashem," he wrote, "are the pictures of my family, if only circumstances had been a little different."

Yad Vashem was an emotional experience for me as well, but I did not connect with it in the same way. Yes, I had met a few Holocaust survivors, most notably Leah Binstock, a cousin who had survived Auschwitz and quietly displayed the numbers on her arm when asked. But, as many historians have noted, as late as the mid-1970s, public discussion of Hitler's massacre of the Jews was muted. For example, I do not recall ever studying it in any great depth in either my European history classes at Hawken School or Hebrew school. When my sister's school, Cleveland Heights High School, offered a class on the Holocaust beginning around 1980, it was said to be one of the first of its kind. So as a teenager who had not lived through World War II and did not yet comprehend the enormity of what had happened, I was somewhat detached. My keen interest in the Holocaust actually emerged once I formally began studying the history of medicine and bioethics and learned about the horrific experiments done by Nazi doctors on Jews at Auschwitz and other concentration camps.

Iran was equally amazing. I would have probably appreciated it even more had I known that visiting the country from the United States would become impossible after the 1979 revolution that ousted the shah. Our most intense outing was to the ruins of Persepolis, which had served as the ancient capital during the years 500 to 300 BC and had been invaded by Alexander the Great. We eventually settled in Shiraz, a southern city that housed the medical school at which my father was teaching. As was to be expected, the American infectious diseases specialist and his son were treated almost like royalty by their hosts. On his first day, my dad diagnosed a rare condition, tuberculosis of the skin, by reviewing a patient's slides himself. He spent his mornings lecturing, and we traveled to various tourist sites in the afternoons.

My father had some trepidation about my returning home by myself. After all, Iran, while a staunch ally of the United States, was an Islamic country, and I was a Jewish teenager flying alone. But the trip through Israel and New York was uneventful. When I arrived in Cleveland on April 9, one of the first things I asked about was Meyer's surgery. My mother told me it had gone well and that he was recuperating in the hospital. I called him, told him all about my trip, and announced that it was completely unacceptable that he and Pearl had never been to Israel. He promised me that they would go. I later learned that he meant it, and had in fact told Pearl later that day that they were going to get passports as soon as he was well.

The phone rang very early the next morning, which was Easter Sunday. My mother answered it. It was my father's brother, Allan. I heard my mother scream and I ran out into the hall. Then, she told me: "Grandpa just died." I remember us hugging and crying.

It was horrible. He was only sixty-nine years old and healthy. I had just spoken with him hours before. My father was thousands of miles away and we had no way to get in touch with him; we had to wait until his planned call that evening.

I had seen the place—long before the era of the cell phone—where my father was going to make the call. It was a public phone located in a communications center in downtown Shiraz. From there, one had to connect with Tehran and reach an international operator. We had done this, with much difficulty, when we first got to Shiraz. The room was chaotic as people waited their turn to use the phone.

When the call came, my mother answered. It was not a great connection. My father asked several times if I had arrived home safely. My mother told him yes, I was fine. She tried to get my father's attention. "Phil," she said, "I have some bad news. Dad died. Dad died." Allan, who was at our house, then took the phone from her and gave him the medical details.

My father later told me what happened after he got off the phone. Another American, waiting to use the phone, realized he was shaken and asked if he was okay. But after that, my dad headed back alone to the small apartment that I had shared with him two days before.

It is Jewish custom to bury the dead as quickly as possible, and my father briefly contemplated staying in Iran and finishing up his teaching duties. But then he changed his mind and decided to return, hoping that the funeral might be delayed and that he would be able to get home in time. Finding a flight from Iran to Cleveland on such short notice, of course, was not easy. Eventually, he made it to Tehran. From there, he was able to get on a flight to John F. Kennedy Airport in New York via London.

My father dealt with his grief by writing. "I feel so placid, calm—certainly in shock," he wrote after packing. "Dad, walk through that door! Please walk through that door." Although my father had been writing to my sister and me on our birthdays, this type of spontaneous rumination on a particular day's events—and the memories they engendered—was different. He would continue to write such entries in notebooks and on yellow legal pads for the next thirty years.

On the plane, my dad could not concentrate enough to read. "I can't cry. I'm not even sad. I'm just objective." He suspected he would let loose when he saw my mother, sister, and me at the airport.

My father did make it back in time for the funeral. The night before, he went to see the body and say good-bye. "He could not have looked more beautiful or restful," he wrote, and he cried a little bit. "The day I'd dreaded for so very long—that moment was suddenly here." Meyer, he mused, would never see another Passover. It would now be up to my father, despite his lack of religious inclinations, to lead the family seder. In three short years, two generations of Lerner men had died, and he was now the eldest.

Interestingly, although I vividly remember talking to Meyer and the early-morning phone call, I have no memory at all of my father's return or of the funeral. I was certainly jet-lagged and emotionally exhausted as well. My father realized that the shock to my system was perhaps even greater than the one to his. "Barron seems to be handling it well—maybe too well," he wrote. For good and for bad, this ability to hold it together in the face of illness and death—what William Osler called "imperturbability"—would persist once I became a doctor. My dad sought me out after the funeral for a walk around the block and told me that we both had to let our emotions come out. This was easier said than done, given our similarly stoic personalities. Indeed, even though it was his father who had died, he was very much playing doctor to the other people affected by Meyer's death. "Must not give into this," he wrote. "Too many people depend on me. I must be strong and stronger." We held the traditional Jewish period of mourning (shivah) at our house and I recall seeing a large number of people from the old Eddy Road neighborhood I had probably never met before. Legions of relatives and friends came to pay their respects.

As with all deaths, my grandpa Meyer's took a while to sink in. I missed him terribly. As the Cleveland Indians began another year of futility, I could not believe we would never again go to a game together. Fortunately, my grandma Pearl was a strong woman and held up pretty well. She certainly had a huge amount of support from her sons, their families, and her large clan of relatives.

My father took the death harder than anyone, playing it over and over in his head. Every time he thought of it, it was like a *zetz* (punch) to the heart. His chest actually "ached." "Going to haunt me, haunt me," he wrote. At one point, he reported having "cracking up thoughts." Meyer had actually had a hernia repaired on the other side a few weeks before the final operation and had done fine. In doing a postoperative check, the surgeon had discovered the second hernia. My father wondered if, in fact, the second hernia had been there all along. If so, Meyer should have had only one operation to fix both of them. If that had happened, he might not have died.

At times, my father tried to view the tragedy as fate—that, for whatever reason, it had been Meyer's time. Although he did not believe in a God, he nevertheless found himself asking, "Why did He put me in Iran now? Why Dad now? Why like this? Why at 5 AM? Why after first Israel visit?" Maybe, my dad reflected, he and I had been Meyer's surrogates in Israel, making the trip that fate (or God) would not let him take.

But my father also believed that he was at least partially to blame, "a key villain" in a preventable death. He never forgave himself for urging his father to get the second operation over with while he was away, especially given Meyer's history of bad veins. Surely, my dad thought, had he been around, he would have done something to

prevent the formation of the blood clot or would have found it earlier and begun treatment to dissolve it. And perhaps the clot formed
because Meyer had undergone two operations in such a short time.
"Did I do it somehow?" he asked. "I can accept the inevitable but
not the accidental."

Was there any basis for his guilt? It is impossible to know, especially since my grandma Pearl had said no to an autopsy. But it
is most likely that my grandfather was the victim of bad luck. All
those involved in the second operation presumably did the same
things they had done before, during, and after the first successful
hernia operation. But this time a known complication of surgery
occurred. My father even admitted this to himself on occasion. "I
know objectively that my being here would've made no difference
whatsoever," he wrote in 1978, "but I keep wondering over and
over, nonetheless."

Another disappointment was to follow, one that may have had
a longer-lasting impact than the death itself: the surgeon who had
done the hernia operation never personally expressed his condolences. There had been a brief opportunity for him to do so, when
my dad returned to the hospital after the period of mourning and
the surgeon was in the same corridor. "I saw him spot me," my father later wrote, "hesitate briefly, then continue on his way, without
a word then, or anytime thereafter."

One can speculate as to why the surgeon did what he did. Losing
the father of his colleague had to have caused the surgeon tremendous guilt. Perhaps he thought my father would reproach him. But
what my dad really wanted was for him to be a good doctor and offer
a warm, human gesture even at the most difficult of times. In retrospect, this event was one of the first of a series of major disappoint-
ments that gradually punctured the idyllic vision of medicine that had
characterized my father's early career. Over the years, he mentioned
it frequently in his journals as something that continued to bother
him. And, in 2006, upon learning that I one day planned to write
this book, he mentioned Meyer's death—and the surgeon's averted
glance—as among the most important events for me to discuss.

In addition to his misgivings about allowing the surgery to proceed while he was away, my father also regretted never having "had the opportunity to repay [Meyer] for the fortunate way our lives turned out." Years later, after seeing a play, *The Loman Family Picnic*, about a struggling working-class family, my father pondered how the uncomplaining Meyer surely must have chafed at spending his whole life as a salaried employee of others.

After the funeral, my dad penned a simple obituary: "Meyer. Born in Poland. Lived and worked in America. Prospered but not in the material sense. We always had food and shelter and essentials. Raised a family, had grandchildren and love from all." But his real tribute to his father was this: every day for a year after Meyer died, either my father or his brother, Allan, two very nonobservant Jews, went to temple to say the Mourner's Kaddish. I went occasionally. Although my father perhaps did this out of a sense of guilt, and although he again found the prayers and rituals "fruitless" and "misleading," he nevertheless persevered because *his* father believed that Judaism was so important. It also kept Meyer "more alive" in his mind, as did looking at his father's driver's license, which my dad had placed in his own wallet, and rubbing his watch, which he kept in a drawer in his office. Going to temple also provided him with serenity and relaxation. The year of Kaddishes began the day after the funeral, and my father, sitting at home, put a yarmulke on his head and tried to learn the whole mourner's prayer so he wouldn't be "faking all but the few well-known first lines." He also mused during the year about resurrecting the huge family seder, inviting all his Cleveland cousins, but this never occurred.

My father's diaries post-1977 contain several entries about Meyer, often in the form of dreams he had about him. For example, on Easter Sunday in April 1987, even though my father had not consciously realized that it was the tenth anniversary of his father's death, he dreamed that Meyer emerged from a swinging door, which caused my dad to awaken with a start. In the dream, Meyer was much younger than he had been when he died, probably in his fifties. Later that day, when my mother pointed out the anniversary and said that she was going to light a Jewish memorial (*yahrzeit*) candle for him, my father actually cried.

In January 1995, my dad woke up from a dream screaming. This time, Meyer had "sauntered around a corner" and frightened him because Meyer was "supposed to be dead." Later that week, my father made the connection. The day before his dream, my son, Ben, almost two years old, had uneventfully undergone correction of two hernias, the same type of operation that had "killed" Meyer. Nonetheless, my father was happy for the visit. "The subconscious is a wondrous thing," he concluded.

It is said that physicians—even those who know the latest statistics from large clinical studies—make many medical decisions based on previous vivid experiences. Such cases tend to be either great saves or bad screwups. I don't know if my father became fixated on preventing blood clots as a result of what happened to Meyer. He was an infectious diseases consultant, so it was not really his bailiwick. Yet even though I was almost a decade away from becoming a doctor when Meyer died, I remained—and still remain—almost obsessive about preventing blood clots. Thus, when I attend on the wards, I regularly scour the list of doctors' orders to make sure that the resident physicians have given patients anticoagulants, compression stockings, or some other appropriate intervention. Have I prevented any blood clots, and perhaps deaths, through my surveillance? Once again, it is impossible to know. But I always felt that my surveillance was a sort of gift that the kind Meyer was giving to his grandson's patients.

We were slowly recovering from Meyer's death when, two months later, my mother found a lump in her left breast. She was only forty-two years old. For the first years in Cleveland, my mom had been a housewife, but once my sister and I were old enough to take care of ourselves, she became bored. Rather than simply returning to the classroom as a teacher, she got interested in educational theory, particularly the idea of tailoring education to fit the student. Eventually, she took courses at a local college, studying learning disabilities. By the mid-1970s, she was teaching children with learning problems in various classroom settings.

I know that my father was proud of what my mother was doing. But his job—and personality—continued to take precedence in the house. My mother was a quiet but strong person, something I would soon come to appreciate even more. But much of her energies went toward placating my father and trying to make him happy while bearing most of the burden of raising my sister and me. Yet when she became sick, it went without saying that my father would assume complete charge of her care.

My memories of my mother being diagnosed with breast cancer are, again, incomplete. I remember my father reassuring all of us that the biopsy of her lump was likely to be negative. I'm not sure if the breast surgeon told him that, or if he thought that himself, or if he was just being his usual paternalistic self, but years later, as a doctor trained in bioethics, I would struggle with this same issue with my own patients. Was it better to be as frank as possible with bad news or to sugarcoat things and always maintain some optimism?

Anyway, I had believed my father enough that when the biopsy came back positive, I was surprised. He told me in the backyard. My mother was inside. I remember hugging him for a long time and then going inside and hugging my mom. Not surprisingly, my mother was much more concerned about the impact of her illness on her family than she was about herself. She reassured me that everything was going to be all right, and I desperately wanted to believe her. Truth be told, the whole experience was a little surreal. I had grown all too familiar with death in the previous few years, but not deaths among members of my parents' generation. I probably could not even conceptualize the possibility of my mother dying.

One great thing about being part of a physician's family is that you have access to very good doctors and are often treated like a VIP. This was especially true in the 1970s, when insurance coverage was less complicated and there was still professional courtesy. My mother's doctor was Charles A. Hubay, a well-respected surgeon at University Hospital, the main teaching hospital of Case Western Reserve. She received the standard operation for the era, a modified radical mastectomy. Because it was 1977, my mother benefited from the activism of women like Rose Kushner. The biopsy and mastectomy were done separately. The modified radical procedure meant that her chest-wall muscles remained intact, which was a much less disfiguring operation than the old Halsted version. Still, my father termed the operation "mutilating" when documenting my mother's ordeal.

The results of my mother's mastectomy showed that the cancer had already spread to two of the underarm lymph nodes located adjacent to the left breast. Moreover, there were also what my father called "emboli" of cancer located higher in the underarm area. Thankfully, there was no evidence of spread to other areas of her body, such as the lungs, liver, brain, and bones. My mother's case was classified as stage II breast cancer because there was disease in the breast and underarm. Once she completed surgery, she received radiation to her chest wall, followed by chemotherapy—powerful intravenous drugs designed to kill any microscopic cancer cells that remained in her body. For the chemotherapy, Hubay entered my mother in a clinical trial that compared various treatments.

It is difficult to conceive of a woman who gets breast cancer in her forties as lucky. But my mother was. First, had she developed cancer only a few years before, she would not have been offered chemotherapy and would likely have died when the invisible areas of cancer grew into metastases. Prophylactic chemotherapy for microscopic disease, which is now routine, had only recently been introduced. Second, she was randomized to the most active arm of Hubay's trial, receiving not only three chemotherapeutic agents but tamoxifen, an anti-estrogen compound, and the Bacillus Calmette-Guérin (BCG) vaccination, designed to boost the patient's immune system. Although BCG turned out to have no salutary effects, tamoxifen decreased recurrences in women who had estrogen-receptor-positive cancers.

Even though Shirley Temple Black, Betty Ford, and Happy Rockefeller had courageously come out about their breast cancers in the five years preceding my mother's diagnosis, secrecy still surrounded the disease. My memories of this time are that things around the house were very hush-hush. My parents surely told our close relatives and friends, but my sister and I were probably instructed to tell people who asked only that my mother was sick.

I don't remember my mother mentioning Betty Ford, but she did read a book written by the journalist Betty Rollin about her experiences with breast cancer. Entitled *First, You Cry*, Rollin's book explicitly avoided what she termed a Pollyanna approach to the disease. Crying, she told her readers, was okay. So, moreover, was laughing. Rollin's book was filled with self-deprecating asides and amusing anecdotes, such as her attempts to find a prosthetic breast at a "tit shop."

But Rollin, who I interviewed for *The Breast Cancer Wars*, was the exception to the rule. As was the case with most women, my mother did not find breast cancer a laughing matter at all. It did not help that the wife of one of my father's boyhood friends was dying of breast cancer at this very same time. On the day the woman died, the husband had frantically called our house, hoping to ask my dad a question about whether he could give morphine to his wife. The man, of course, had no idea about my mom's recent diagnosis, but it is hard to imagine a more jarring event for someone battling the same disease.

I recall my mother spending a huge amount of time by herself in her bedroom. She had never been a person who tolerated medications well, and what my father called her "god-damn chemo" consisted of considerably higher doses of the three agents in question—Cytoxan, methotrexate, and 5-fluorouracil—than are given today. In the early era of chemotherapy for an often fatal disease, it was assumed that more was better. In addition, the medications available for the side effects of chemotherapy, notably nausea, were not especially effective. I remember hearing a lot of retching and vomiting coming from behind her closed door. The treatment induced early menopause, leading to hot flashes. Regrettably, my frugal and self-abnegating parents did not install air-conditioning to help relieve her symptoms during another humid Cleveland summer. My father speculated that the experimental BCG immunotherapy my mother received probably added to her discomfort by causing rheumatoid arthritis–like pain in her joints.

I recall being mildly irritated with her, wishing at times that she might try a little harder. I suspect that, as a teenager, I wanted my mother to be as normal as possible. In retrospect, I see that her response to the disease was an example of my mother's strength. She had been diagnosed with a potentially fatal disease in an era in which a diagnosis of breast cancer came with shame and stigma. Plus, she had suffered greatly from her treatment. Her extensive time by herself was a primary part of a stiff-upper-lip mentality that enabled her to deal with the vicissitudes of her illness.

Along these lines, I do not remember there being many visitors at our house during my mother's treatment. To the best of my recollection, we mostly managed on our own, relying on my grandmothers to help out with meals and with getting my sister and me off to school. Indeed, during the first couple of years of my mother's illness, several people who were friends with her or with both of my parents dropped off the radar screen. Overtly, at least, my mother was not resentful, speculating that her diagnosis of potentially fatal breast cancer at age forty-two had probably just overwhelmed them. Still, it had to hurt. In later years, when my father had advanced Parkinson's disease, and the number of visitors to the house again seemed smaller than it should have been, I revisited what had happened decades earlier. My parents are extremely private by nature and it is quite possible that in some instances, my mother, inadvertently or not, had gently pushed people away. As late as December 1978, they canceled a New Year's Eve party at our house because my mom was simply not up to it.

My father, of course, was a rock. He was caregiver, reassurer, and all-controlling presence for his patients, and these tendencies became magnified when the patient was his wife. "Thank God, I can be strong here," he wrote nine days after the mastectomy. "I must steel myself, strengthen myself and protect her as best I can," he added. "And protect the others as well." His paternalist inclinations were present in full force. Concealing the cancer diagnosis from my mother, which he might have tried to do ten or twenty years earlier, was certainly no longer an option. But doling out selected bits and pieces of information to various family members, including my mom herself, most surely was. For example, the only person my dad informed about the cancer emboli was his brother, since Allan was also a doctor. "I can't tell her about the emboli," he wrote, "because I don't know their significance." (Years later, when I had joined the fraternity of doctors, he told me about them. I was interested to learn the details but I responded, predictably, by questioning all the secrecy, something that doctors were no longer supposed to do. I asked him if he had ever told my mother about the emboli, and he said no.) While my father remained publicly optimistic about the chemotherapy, in private he was not so sure. "Does the chemo cure or just delay?" he asked himself. "When can we breathe easily? Three years maybe, but I don't know." When reading my dad's journals, I found an even more perplexing example of how he had micromanaged things: at one point, he ordered a blood test on her to check for residual cancer and speculated that he would not tell anyone if it was positive.

Did my mother suspect that her doctor-husband was protecting her from bad news? I'm not sure, but it probably did not occur to her to ask. My father could be imperious, and, occasionally, my mom challenged his authority. But when it came to his role as physician, she ceded almost all control. It is hard to imagine a doctor's wife doing otherwise in the 1970s.

If my father withheld information in public, he profusely confided to his journals, not only about my mother's disease and its prognosis, but also about the enormous emotional impact it was having on him. "Cancer is a hard, ugly word," he wrote on June 15, 1977, the day of her diagnosis. As a physician, he well knew what lay ahead, "how changed our lives will soon become." This week "we join the ranks of the 'someone else' it always happens to," he perceptively noted. "I don't want to lose my wife, my life. Can this really be happening to me?" In another entry, he wrote: "If I should lose her, what could there be for me after that? I tremble with fear, even to contemplate such a terror."

When my father first learned the biopsy results, with the positive lymph nodes and emboli, he wrote, "Today I found out I'll not have her for very long." My dad's devotion to the scientific basis of medicine left him with little interest in religion or the supernatural. But my mother's diagnosis threatened to change this. "Sudden thunder and a storm as I write the word 'metastasis,'" he remarked one Saturday afternoon.

The next crisis came in March 1978, when my mother discovered a bump along her mastectomy scar. It was hard not to fear the worst. Scars are a common place for breast cancers to recur. My mother again saw Charles Hubay, who removed the tissue and sent it to the pathology laboratory for analysis. Then it was time to wait. On the first night, my father took my sister to temple "for company" as he prayed for his father. The next night, my mother actually made a rare appearance there. The next day, my dad admitted to himself (only) that he was "quite terrified" and had "lost almost all control." He called Hubay's office to see if the result was back but the staff did not know. Then he decided to use his trump card, his MD degree. He called the pathology laboratory at University Hospital himself and found a doctor who was able to provide extremely good news: it was merely a stitch abscess, a small area of infection. "Relief is not the word," my father wrote. "Flowed, gushed, overwhelmed is more like it."

Reading my father's words was poignant for me. Although he had done what he could to ensure that my mother would receive excellent care, beyond that, the situation was out of his control. Whether my mom lived or died would depend on her doctors, the treatments they recommended, and, to a large degree, good or bad luck. Yet staying in control—or appearing to—was what my father believed he needed to do, for his own sake and for others'. So he controlled what he could: information. This was full-fledged paternalism. And while it was understandable, given both my father's profession and his personality, it was also a burden for him.

My dad allowed himself a little more relaxation on November 8, 1978. It was my parents' twentieth wedding anniversary and they went to Charley's Crab, their favorite special-occasion restaurant. Fortunately, Phil had remembered to order flowers; in this case, twenty red roses. My mother was not feeling great and she was hardly out of the woods. But they were at a nice restaurant and celebrating. And my mother was even quietly contemplating the possibility of breast reconstruction. As fate would have it, that same evening, CBS aired what my father termed a "not bad" made-for-television adaptation of the Betty Rollin book *First, You Cry*, starring Mary Tyler Moore. My parents dutifully watched it together, although my father felt my mother "tightening" and "shuddering" as the "similar stories unfolded."

Phil Lerner may have been doing a pretty good job of managing his wife's cancer, but, ironically, his professional life suddenly felt less fulfilling. Meyer's death and my mother's cancer, I learned from his journals, delivered a one-two punch from which he never really recovered. Only days after my grandfather's death, my father suddenly felt at sea, undirected. Among those who had come to Meyer's shivah was my grandma Pearl's sister Shirley, who had experienced a major stroke and was in "undeserved" pain—both physical and emotional.

"It should have been me," she told my father.

"She's right, of course," he wrote later that day. "How she is suffering." He then speculated as to whether the stroke had affected her brain or unmasked previously concealed anger and angst.

But then he abruptly dropped the subject. "It's reached the point when I'm tired of questions because surely there are no answers," he wrote. "At least they elude me. And I usually have all the answers."

As a man of medicine, my father knew as well as anyone how random and unfair illness could be. He had certainly seen enough patients and family members die far too young and seen others survive for far too long. Until this point, however, he had been able to use his clinical judgment and professional connections to influence or at least ameliorate these situations. But now he felt helpless. His essentially healthy father had died unnecessarily while he was thousands of miles away. Meanwhile, Aunt Shirley and so many others like her went on living despite chronic misery. As he had with my mother, my dad got Shirley excellent physicians and offered good medical advice to her. But he saw these as trivial interventions compared with her overall health, which was so poor. When he returned to the hospital after Meyer's funeral, two of the first patients he saw as the infectious diseases consult had advanced, recurrent cancers. "What's to save?" he asked. "Why prolong the agony?"

Indeed, in the days after the funeral, my father had dreaded going back to work—something that had never happened before. Part of it, presumably, was the exhaustion after what he had just been through. Part of it was having to treat patients with such dismal prognoses without being able to save the Meyer Lerners of the world. But his ennui even extended to his research, which was the intellectual engine that had always kept him going, night after night. "Will I recover energy, want to tackle a big paper again?" he asked himself in May 1977. "Right now, can't even dream of it."

What was going on here? Perhaps, my father wrote in one entry, it was depression. But his journals contained a revelation that surprised me. My dad's working-class childhood had led to his determination to succeed, but his fanatical devotion to medicine and sick patients had specifically been his way of thanking and paying back his family, especially Meyer, who had never had the chance to achieve his own dreams. On the one-year anniversary of Meyer's death, my father penned him a note saying how much he missed him, writing that "so much of what I did and do, I did unconsciously to give you *naches*" (special joy). Years later, when my dad applied to be promoted from an associate professor to a full professor, he did it "mostly for Meyer." But with Meyer no longer alive, things had changed. "I think," my father concluded, "that's why the zest is gone."

My mother's illness only compounded the inertia and soul-searching. In April 1978, my father remarked that she had only two more cycles of chemotherapy and he hoped that when it was over, the weight on his shoulders would be lifted. Putting together the infectious diseases syllabus for the medical students, a task in which he had once reveled, was now "like pulling teeth." At one point he even confessed that he was doing just enough to get by, the cardinal sin that he so often condemned in others, including me.

Then, in late October 1978, my father began to experience palpitations in his chest, accompanied, at times, by what he called heartburn. He was worried enough to see a cardiologist, who ordered a stress test. When that was inconclusive, he underwent a cardiac catheterization in December 1978. The test revealed a significant blockage of a branch of one of his coronary arteries. There were no other problems and no evidence of a past heart attack, but there were enough worrisome findings for my father to announce to himself: "I am now officially a cardiac patient."

Like so many other physicians and laypeople who learn that they have heart disease, my dad treated the news as a wake-up call: "If I get my weight down, keep it down, keep [blood pressure] down, get cholesterol down and learn to live a little more relaxed, I wonder if I can't reverse that *one* damn narrowing." Even after he received this news, however, my father remained a classic yo-yo dieter, alternating periods of abstinence and substantial weight loss with regular nighttime raids on the refrigerator. He was also a familiar face at the Department of Medicine's weekly Friday-afternoon GI Rounds, where he enjoyed mingling with the house staff but also ate more than his share of the free food.

Not surprisingly, the heart episode was largely carried out in secret—even the catheterization. My father told his physician-brother but not me or my mother, whom he deemed too fragile due to her cancer and ongoing treatment. "I'm totally unafraid of death at the moment," he confided in a journal entry. Reading this phrase stirred a memory of my forty-six-year-old father announcing to me, right around this time, that he had lived a long and full life and it would not be so terrible if he died. In retrospect, this was probably his way of telling his son that he had a heart condition and might not be around forever—without actually saying that. I suspect it was also his way of alleviating my guilt if something bad were to happen— exactly what Meyer had never had the chance to do for him.

Stories like this are great fodder for biographical memoirs, but I wish he had just told me the truth at the time. I recall spending a lot of time scratching my head about his statement and was probably a little freaked out. It is another reminder of how paternalistic behavior, while well meaning, may have unforeseen negative consequences. Incidentally, although my father had numerous medical problems over the years, his heart apparently remained fine, even though his efforts at eating better and exercising more were always transient. So much for willpower.

The events of 1977 and 1978—Meyer's unexpected death, my mother's cancer, and my father's heart blockage—cast a major pall over my dad's life. "The pendulum has certainly swung with a vengeance," he wrote. "My charmed life is now balancing out with a bang."

And even though these events were as much bad luck as a failure of the medical system, my father seemed to feel that somehow medicine had let him down. That same field that had given him so much—a path out of East Cleveland, intellectual stimulation, professional status, and a way to channel his gratitude to his family—was now taking much away from him, and threatening to take away more.

I had been giving serious thought to becoming a doctor since I first began to volunteer at the Montefiore Home. The events of 1977, while leading my father to feel disenchanted with medicine, conversely fostered my interest in following in his footsteps, although I would not realize this connection until several years later.

I was sure enough about my potential career choice that, when I matriculated at the University of Pennsylvania in September 1978, I signed up for inorganic chemistry, biology, and calculus. I was officially a premed.

CHAPTER FOUR

The Second Dr. Lerner

These days, it is common for future doctors to take off a year or more at some point during their training—before, after, or even during medical school. This time off enables them to see the world, have a real job, or simply take a break. In my era, such gaps were uncommon, and I, like my father, was a straight arrow.

Thus, from September 1978, when I began college, to June 1989, when I completed my residency in internal medicine, I was thoroughly immersed in as intense an educational process as one could imagine. In retrospect, it almost seems like that amusement-park ride in which a small railcar makes sharp turns and jerks the passenger from side to side before suddenly emerging into the light. But I was also identifying those aspects of medicine—such as bioethics, history, and the doctor-patient relationship—that I would eventually combine with my clinical work.

This decade would be a momentous time not only for me, but for medicine. As I went onto the wards for the first time, in the early 1980s, all the talk seemed to be about two diseases—one old and one new. Tuberculosis, which I associated with the abandoned Sunny Acres sanatorium my father once showed me in Cleveland, had roared back, and we did not even have proper isolation rooms for patients. The hospital and the medical profession were even more unprepared to deal with the acquired immunodeficiency syndrome, a baffling new infectious disease that destroyed patients' immune systems and then killed them. Those of us caring for these patients had a sense that we were living history, and we were.

My decision to attend the University of Pennsylvania was almost random. For reasons I cannot remember, I never considered applying to small liberal arts colleges, only to large universities located in cities. Penn was one of these, and adding it to my list was practically an afterthought. I made a quick stop there and took a one-hour campus tour while on my way to Baltimore to visit Johns Hopkins, where two of my best friends, a year older than I, were freshmen. Since college is a time to make new friends and try new things, it was fortunate that I did not get accepted to Hopkins. When I looked at my range of offers in the spring of 1978, Penn it was. I did not go back for another visit before deciding.

Considering that I had gone to a tiny suburban private high school, my transition to a large university in a big city was relatively smooth. My proposed plan of study probably helped. I was a premedical student and planned to major in American history, so there were a lot of required courses for me to take.

Not everybody approved of my plan. In the late 1970s, it was customary for premeds to major in one of the sciences, which presumably matched their career interests and evidenced a devotion to science. I remember a few people who thought that being a history major might count against me when I applied to medical school. Fortunately, I stuck to my guns.

One thing that had changed for me was my diligence. Ironically, perhaps, away from my father's disapproving gaze, I decided to work extremely hard in my classes. Although I did write for the school newspaper, play in every intramural softball or basketball game I could, go to some parties, and hang out with my friends, I could be found most often in the library. Why this change? Part of it had to do with a latent competitiveness. Attending classes with other premeds who, I felt, were often cutthroat, I wanted to do better than them. And by the end of the first month of school, I knew that I could. In retrospect, I think that Hawken, where my grades had been up and down, prepared me incredibly well for college. After having taken the equivalent of AP chemistry, physics, biology, and calculus in high school, I found that the material was relatively easy if I studied hard enough.

Although I insisted on merging history and medicine as an undergraduate, I remained remarkably uninformed about the combination. Penn's history department housed two of the country's preeminent historians of medicine, Charles Rosenberg and Rosemary Stevens, but it never occurred to me to take their classes. The union of my interests finally came about due to chance and good luck. As a senior history major, I needed to write an honors thesis. My professor, Walter Licht, a labor historian, proposed that, as a future doctor, I consider a medical topic. I said okay but had no ideas at all. Licht suggested that I visit the university's archives and see if the staff there might help.

So it was that I first realized the truth of the phrase "The archivist is the historian's best friend." Archives director Francis Dallett told me about a missionary medical school begun by Penn in China in 1905, the story of which had never been told. There were lots of relevant primary materials both at Penn and at other universities. I was off to the races. I loved doing the research, going through aged and fragile documents in reading rooms and taking notes on what turned out to be thousands of small note cards. I needed an adviser, and so it was that I finally met Charles Rosenberg, who claimed to know little about the topic but was of course an enormous help.

Meanwhile, I was applying to medical school. If my father had become a doctor in part as a way to give back to his industrious and frugal working-class parents and relatives who had made so many sacrifices for him, my decision stemmed from being raised in a comfortable liberal upper-middle-class home with two parents who explicitly modeled ethical behavior: my father, the compassionate and devoted physician, and my mother, a remarkably selfless person whose bout with and recovery from breast cancer led her to become an inveterate volunteer for the American Cancer Society—eventually even winning an award as Cleveland's top volunteer of the year. That is, I pursued medicine not as a way to acknowledge my good fortune or surmount personal odds but rather as a way to do good for others. As someone with an interest in history and the humanities, I added an intellectual component to my career: scrutiny of the very profession that I had chosen to join. My father had entered medicine wide-eyed, but I entered it with my eyes open to the complicated and controversial issues that came with the territory.

I suppose that the topic of my honors thesis did arise during some of my medical school interviews, but at the time, I was planning to become a doctor, not a historian. Having compiled an impressive academic record, I was invited for a large number of interviews. First up was—no surprise—Case Western Reserve School of Medicine, my father's alma mater and employer. My father had not suggested that I attend college in Cleveland, but medical school was a different story. So I had applied to Case's medical school, even though we both knew I would probably not wind up there. We arranged for me to have the interview at the end of August 1981, just before I left Cleveland to return to Philadelphia for my senior year.

I can only begin to imagine how proud my father was that day when we entered the office of Jack Caughey, the iconoclastic (then emeritus) admissions director who had accepted my father to the same school twenty-five years earlier and who had played a major role in curricular reform. The interview was, of course, a formality. There was no chance that Professor Phillip Lerner's son, who had compiled an excellent record and was—perfect for Case—a history major, would not be offered admission. My father and I also paid a visit to the University of Michigan Medical School. I was amused, years later, to read in my father's journals that he had been "infuriated" that my only interviewer there had been a medical student, an issue that had not even occurred to me.

Another early interview took place at the Columbia College of Physicians and Surgeons in October 1981, during (as I recall) the school's first week of interviews. I liked the idea of going to New York City for medical school, and Columbia was certainly prestigious. But before the meeting, I walked around the rather dreary Washington Heights neighborhood in which the school was situated, and it was not love at first sight.

An interesting event, however, occurred during my interview. Like other medical school interviewees, I had gotten advice about how to answer some of the questions I would probably be asked on the circuit. So I was prepared to explain why I had applied to medical school, why I had majored in history, what I planned to do during medical school (laboratory research, I dubiously claimed!), and what I might eventually choose as a specialty. But I was caught completely off guard by one of the questions asked by my interviewer, a faculty psychiatrist.

"What," he asked, "was the most difficult thing you have ever experienced in your life?" I paused for a moment, thinking about my answer. But there was little question what it would be: my mother's breast cancer. I wish I could remember exactly what I said but I do recall the words and feelings pouring out of me. The fact was that, although my family had often discussed the cancer, there had been no *real* conversations of the sort that my father was having with himself in his journal. So it was that I first openly expressed my fears that my mother was going to die in an interview room at Columbia. The discussion also helped crystallize in my mind why I had chosen to apply to medical school: to help sick patients like my mother.

The interviewer must have realized that he had not received a cookie-cutter answer. Within a couple of weeks, a fat envelope arrived in my college mailbox offering me admission to Columbia. But I was not done interviewing. I made a lot of other trips, including one to Harvard Medical School. My father had insisted that I look up his old mentor Louis Weinstein, who I had not seen since we moved from Boston to Cleveland fifteen years earlier. We had a nice chat in his large, cluttered office at Harvard's Brigham and Women's Hospital, where he had moved after leaving Tufts. I remember being impressed with his vast knowledge, just as my dad had been during their chance encounter in 1960. So I decided to mention to my tour guide, a Harvard medical student, that I had met with the venerable professor. His reply was not what I expected. "Weinstein." He sighed. "He just goes on and on about those old diseases like tuberculosis." I felt a little embarrassed at having mentioned Weinstein, but I later took solace in the fact that as the student and

I were speaking, the tuberculosis bacterium was quietly planning a major resurgence.

By early 1982, I had completed my interviews. Once I heard back from all the schools, I considered my options. Columbia, I decided, was the place where I would become a doctor.

On the one hand, it is amazing that my father did not move me into medical school in August 1982. After all, having his son become a doctor was something he had dreamed about for years. I remember any number of fathers (and mothers) carrying boxes into Columbia's Bard Hall, the residence for most first-year P&S (shorthand for Columbia College of Physicians and Surgeons) students. On the other hand, his absence was utterly explicable. He was tending to his uncle Mickey, his father's youngest brother, who was dying of cancer. My dad visited him daily, providing advice about pain relief, answering medical questions, and simply sitting with him for long periods. Certainly no one would have begrudged my father's going to New York for a few days—even if Mickey had died while he was away. After all, something momentous was occurring, and Mickey surely had other doctors. But he stayed and, indeed, was at the bedside when Mickey quietly died, the same day that I departed. For reasons I cannot remember, my mother stayed in Cleveland as well.

This is a somewhat painful anecdote for me to revisit, as, once again, it seems, my father had put being a doctor over being a parent. But I do not recall being very upset at the time. I knew that my dad was extremely proud of me. And, on the precipice of entering medical school, I surely was inspired by his profound devotion to his dying uncle. So I drove to New York with Toby Nygaard, a neurologist who had done an internal medicine residency in Cleveland at the Mount Sinai and become friendly with my parents. Even though Mickey died later that day, my father was thinking about me. "So tonight Barron is in New York," he wrote, "on the threshold."

My move from high school to college was relatively easy, but the transition to medical school was more difficult. I really enjoyed orientation week, but as soon as classes began, things got very serious very quickly. I remember many of my classmates heading to the library the first evening after classes, something even I had not done in college. And one of our anatomy professors began his first lecture by telling us that if we had not already begun memorizing anatomical structures, we were behind. Meanwhile, as a former history major, I was feeling a little overwhelmed. At least half the class, it seemed, had taken biochemistry—one of our introductory courses—in college. Some of my fellow students had even taken histology, the study of cells and tissues. I did not even know what the word meant.

It was a little unseemly for me to complain about all of this. Just because I had worked so hard in college and now apparently needed a little break did not mean that my classmates felt the same way. But, in my defense, the classwork was particularly tedious, mostly just dry talks about molecules, chemical reactions, and body parts. Compared to these presentations, my father's lectures had been downright exciting.

It was clear why many of the lectures were so uninspiring. Many of the first-year faculty members were basic-science researchers, much more comfortable behind a microscope than in front of a hundred and fifty medical students. Only in later years did I realize that many of these individuals had been giants in their respective fields. Biochemist Elvin A. Kabat, for example, had made some of the most important discoveries about how the body produces the antibodies that attack invading bacteria. Hematologist Elliott Osserman knew more than anyone about two rare diseases involving abnormal proteins: multiple myeloma and amyloidosis. These professors were probably too modest to emphasize their own achievements, but some historical perspective would have made things more interesting—at least for me. I could not resist telling the microbiologist Harold S. Ginsberg, a pioneer in the study of adenoviruses, a bit of his own history: he had taught my father microbiology at Western Reserve University in the 1950s, and now, in the 1980s, he was teaching it to me.

I did have one confidante during my early days at P&S: Evelyn Attia, a classmate who had also been a history major in college and was feeling similarly deluged. The composition of medical schools had changed substantially from my father's era, with its overwhelming predominance of white men. Evelyn was one of about forty women in my class of a hundred and fifty students, and, within a decade, Columbia and most other medical schools would attain a ratio close to fifty-fifty. We also had about twenty minority students. Although I had, in some ways, benefited from being a white male, I appreciated the changes, which brought a diversity of opinions and experiences to the laboratory and the wards. In fact, on several occasions when these women and minority students witnessed behaviors that they believed to be sexist or racist, they confronted the rest of the class. Sad to say, several faculty members held outdated views about gender and race, which they blithely broadcast. We students at times did the same. As a liberal person who had trained in the humanities, I considered myself fairly enlightened, but I was forced to confront some of my own prejudices.

Soon after my arrival at P&S, in a situation that mirrored my father's unexpected and fortunate introduction to Louis Weinstein and the field of infectious diseases, I encountered someone who would become one of my mentors. It occurred in a class called Society and Medicine, which was being offered to P&S medical students for the first time. The lecturer, David J. Rothman, introduced himself as a United States historian from the main campus of Columbia University who had been asked to move to the medical center to study and teach about a new set of ethical issues being raised by technological advances, patient activism, and a spate of recent research scandals.

Most of my classmates did not especially like the course, seeing it as peripheral to becoming a doctor. But I ate up the Society and Medicine syllabus, which introduced me to a series of seminal controversies that defined the field of bioethics in its early years. For example, there was the 1961 article published in the *Journal of the American Medical Association* reporting that 90 percent of physicians preferred not to tell cancer patients their true diagnoses. This attitude stemmed not from any scientific research but the doctors' "emotion-laden *a priori* personal judgments" that patients needed to be protected from bad news. There was the story of the God Squad, a committee of laypeople in Seattle in 1962 who were asked to decide which patients with chronic kidney failure would receive lifesaving hemodialysis from the limited number of available machines. Those left undialyzed would die. When the committee used social-worth criteria, favoring individuals who had families and went to church, the public objected strongly. Another important event was a report published in 1968 by the Harvard Medical School Ad Hoc Committee on Brain Death. This group of thirteen men—mostly physicians—argued that patients who had beating hearts but no electrical activity in the brain should be declared dead, an entirely new concept. Critics, however, argued that this definition of brain death was primarily a mechanism for increasing the number of available transplant organs. While this was a worthwhile cause, they believed, it had the potential to take advantage of dying patients and their vulnerable families.

A substantial amount of class time was spent on Willowbrook, Tuskegee, and the other research scandals of the 1960s and 1970s in which the principle of informed consent had been repeatedly violated. And there was the well-known 1975 Karen Ann Quinlan case, in which a young woman, after ingesting an unknown quantity of pills and alcohol, had become irreversibly comatose. When her parents asked that their daughter be removed from the ventilator that was keeping her alive, the Catholic hospital refused. Eventually, the New Jersey Supreme Court sided with the family, and its ruling helped codify the notion that gravely ill patients had the "right to die." Ironically, when the ventilator was turned off, Quinlan, unexpectedly, lived—still in a coma—for nine more years.

A variety of ethical issues were raised by these episodes, including truth-telling, rationing of scarce resources, informed consent, experimentation, and the rights of the dying. But they all shared a common thread: patients, or, in the case of research, human subjects, were actively excluded from clinical decision making and at times used as a means to an end. My father and other doctors of his generation justified such behavior as beneficent or helpful for the greater good, but the new bioethics found it entirely unacceptable.

After Rothman's first lecture, Evelyn and I approached him and identified ourselves as college history majors. The two of us began to hang out at the Center for the Study of Society and Medicine, which Rothman was running. During the summer between the first and second year of medical school, Evelyn and I did research projects on the history of Presbyterian Hospital, spending most of our time at the archives on the Columbia main campus. It was terrific and very rejuvenating. So were other outside activities that I pursued during medical school. I finally put my ten years of clarinet lessons to use and played in the pit for several surprisingly good musicals performed by a P&S student theater group, the Bard Hall Players. And I became very active in a local organization that opposed American military policies in Central America and sent health supplies to the region. Pursuing these endeavors took time away from my studies but somehow seemed to provide balance and perspective to my nascent career in medicine.

Despite my early dissatisfaction with the curriculum, there were bright spots. In an innovative course called the Physician-Patient Relationship, patients were regularly invited to speak to our class. That it was taught by a general internist named Constance Park underscored the humanistic approach that women physicians could bring to medical education. To show our respect for the patients, we were expected to wear our white coats to these presentations. In one sense, these meetings were a throwback to traditional grand rounds, in which doctors gathered in an amphitheater in their starched white coats and neckties to hear interesting cases and, at times, meet the patients. But they were also a reaction to these earlier sessions in which patients were publicly examined but rarely asked to participate. The first PPR class was a huge eye-opener. The guest was a woman with diabetes who had used a labor-intensive insulin regimen to successfully carry and deliver a healthy baby, thereby countering the long-standing opinion of many medical experts that pregnancy was too risky for diabetic women. She spoke candidly and forcefully about her decisions and experiences. It was one of the few instances—aside from Rothman's course—when we addressed the concept of an empowered patient. Actually meeting one was even better.

Fortunately, classes during my second year were considerably more interesting. Rather than learning simply how the healthy body worked, we were learning pathophysiology—how the body malfunctioned in the case of an enormous range of diseases. Two professors from the division of infectious diseases, Harold C. Neu and Glenda J. Garvey, gave some of the most interesting lectures and often won Best Teacher awards. Neu knew my father very well, and I made sure to go and introduce myself. He apparently said something to Garvey, because when I met her, she was, well, thrilled. "Your dad is the endocarditis Lerner," she immediately announced. Garvey, who ran the all-important internal medicine clerkship for third-year P&S medical students, was one of the most respected woman physicians at the medical center. She would eventually become a good friend and the most important figure in my medical training.

By the summer of 1984, my classmates and I were pretty burned out. We had spent two years memorizing enormous amounts of material and taking test after test. P&S finally put us on the wards for a physical-diagnosis course, in which we interviewed and examined patients. This was my first experience seeing great cases, patients with disorders that had been identified as particularly interesting and thus were ideal for eager medical students to see. I was in a group of five students; we were supervised by one of the veteran internists at the medical center, a man I will call Dr. Jones. Jones was a 1943 graduate of P&S and probably in his mid- to late sixties.

My recollections of this course, plus the first two clinical rotations of my third year, are enhanced by a brief journal that I kept from May to August of 1984. I had largely forgotten about this effort and did not reread the entries until 2012, when I was working on this book. As one might imagine, there were stories in the journals that I remembered and others that I had long since forgotten. On the whole, however, it helps to explain why I chose my subsequent career path.

Although I loved being on the wards, meeting actual patients, and seeing actual pathology, I almost immediately felt uncomfortable with the physical-diagnosis course. Some type of permission was probably obtained for our visits, but it was hard to believe that the patients really knew what they were getting themselves into. Typically, one or two of us would interview and examine the patient.

Later on, we would present our findings to Jones and the rest of the group. Then we would all go back to see the patient. Jones would typically ask a few more questions and then watch as the rest of the students performed an examination. Then we would talk about what we had found, all the while standing around the patient's bed. "The patients," I wrote, "were hardly people to me." I don't recall translating our highly medicalized discussions into comprehensible terms for them nor asking if they had any questions. We generally just thanked the patient, hopefully covered him or her up, and left the room.

Some of this was generational. Physicians of Jones's era were generally comfortable with seeing ward patients as what was called teaching material, patients available to help educate doctors in training in exchange for essentially free care at a major medical center. And this wasn't necessarily all bad. Jones and his patrician contemporaries, many with upscale private practices in midtown Manhattan, oozed confidence, sagacity, and, at times, a lot more empathy than we younger folks. W. Proctor Harvey, a skilled Georgetown University cardiologist who practiced in this era, liked to emphasize the importance of shaking patients' hands and, if necessary, even plumping up their pillows. One of my favorite stories, told by the physician-writer Abigail Zuger in the *New York Times*, described the time that she and her rumpled fellow residents decided to annoy their supervising Park Avenue attending by bringing him to meet a belligerent patient who was refusing to leave the hospital. His white coat, Zuger wrote, "was from another era: snowy thick 100 percent cotton fastened with braided cotton toggles." "Hello dear," the doctor said to the patient, and he cradled her hand in both of his. "Ten minutes later," Zuger remarked, "the two of them were sitting side by side on her bed, making animated plans for her discharge."

Jones, however, was especially behind the times. He still called African Americans "colored." Thus, it was hardly surprising that when we visited a black patient with abdominal pain, Jones's first comments were about how much alcohol the patient had drunk and the fact that he was apparently a drug dealer. Even though I realized that a complete drug and alcohol history was crucial for all patients, regardless of their race, I was concerned that Presbyterian

Hospital physicians were biasing their patient care due to what I termed *preconceived suppositions.* What I did not record was my response to these types of behaviors, which disturbed me and my fellow classmates. As I recall, we rolled our eyes but said nothing to either Jones or the patients. We were, unfortunately, too intimidated by the strict hierarchy in medicine, which discouraged any criticism of one's superiors.

The problem of balancing the care of patients with students' need to learn, which I labeled the *great third-year conflict,* was not limited to rounds with more senior physicians. During one physical-diagnosis session, an internal medicine resident took us on what I called classic medical rounds, whisking us from room to room to examine patients. It was an invaluable teaching experience: I felt my first enlarged liver and heard several different heart murmurs. But it had to have been a jarring experience for the patients. "It doesn't matter if you are napping, about to undergo surgery, or whatever," I wrote. "You will be exposed and examined whenever a mass of white coats congregates at your bedside."

Two specific examples from my notes vividly demonstrate what happened when earnest, and generally polite, doctors had as their primary focus the need to learn. The resident introduced one patient, a young, deaf African American woman, as "Miss Smith, an intravenous drug abuser." Even though that fact may have been true, it was surely a denigrating appellation. As we examined the patient, she writhed around in pain. The resident tried to soothe her, calling her "honey" and "sweetie," but that was unlikely to help someone who was deaf. Of a second patient, a woman with schizophrenia and a swollen abdomen, I felt as if she "had no clue as to who we were or what was going on." As we examined her, she kept trying to cover herself with the sheet. Even the resident was somewhat uncomfortable, remarking that he hated to treat patients as teaching material.

It is not as if P&S was oblivious to this type of issue, as shown by Rothman's and Park's courses. Plus, shortly before the physical-diagnosis course began, the school had offered my class an awareness seminar that discussed issues such as racism, sexism, and homophobia (although, unfortunately, only eighteen of the hundred and fifty students in my class attended). One of the exercises was for the white students to pretend they were minority students and vice versa. But it was one thing for students to discuss respect and equality in the classroom and quite another for them to speak up on the wards if they thought that a patient's dignity was being violated. I confined my thoughts to paper.

Why did I find these issues—the ethics of a teaching hospital, the professional development of medical students, and the need to balance learning with caring—particularly compelling? I suspect that these interests stemmed from the values of my parents, my intellectual attraction to the humanities, and my early, intense exposure to my father's brand of patient-centered medicine. As I would find out, the third and fourth years of medical school and then residency training raised an almost endless source of ethical and philosophical questions.

When I began my third-year clinical rotations in July 1984, I was thrown into the fire, doing obstetrics and gynecology at Harlem Hospital Center. If Presbyterian Hospital was the mecca, an Ivy League–run institution full of high-achieving physicians and fascinating cases referred from all over the country, Harlem, a public hospital, was the safety net for a largely poor African American neighborhood. The quality of the medical and nursing staffs was variable, but there were many extremely talented clinicians who had specifically chosen to work there.

Unfortunately, constant financial pressures meant that Harlem Hospital was always crowded and chaotic. Providing patient-centered care required lots of extra effort. Some staff members went out of their way to comfort and listen to patients, but many did not. The residents who staffed the labor and delivery suite, for example, would go from bed to bed saying, "Push, push, miss!" or "Kaka, kaka, senora." I wrote at the time that the ob-gyn residents, most of whom were women and minorities themselves, did not seem to remember the patients' names. I was also concerned that inadequate amounts of anesthetic were being given to the largely poor and minority patients who were giving birth—and that the particularly annoying patients

seemed a little less heinous. "I was angry at my patients," I admitted. "Yes, it's happened already. And it was directly proportional to my lack of sleep."

The constant workload was difficult for me for two other reasons. First, there was very little time to read about the diseases that I was encountering. Given the choice between reading and sleeping, I preferred to go to sleep. Second, an eighty- to hundred-hour workweek was cramping my style. I had prided myself on maintaining a diversity of interests during the first two years of medical school. But now there was very little time to read the *New York Times*, much less jog, go to the gym, eat out, or engage in political activities. What did it mean that, this early in my career, I was fighting what I called a "maniacal devotion to medicine"? Was I guarding against my father's decision to become so immersed in his career that he neglected other aspects of his life, including his family? Perhaps. But how could I become a patient-centered physician like my father and his generation of doctors without completely focusing on my work?

"Twelve days since I last wrote," I remarked in mid-August, toward the end of the ob-gyn rotation. "I'm afraid the diary has been a casualty to other activities." And so it was. There were two more entries, both during the next rotation, pediatrics, which I did at Babies Hospital back at Columbia. In contrast to obstetrics, with its unpredictability and fast turnover of patients, inpatient pediatrics featured a large number of ongoing, devastating cases. Not surprisingly, I was drawn to the family dynamics and the ethical issues raised by such sad stories. For example, the mother of a boy dying of a rare cancer learned every little scrap of information as a way to try to maintain control of a terrible situation. I entirely sympathized with her but bristled a little when she told him to stop eating gumdrops. *What the hell is the difference?* I thought. Even though I was not especially good at interacting with children, I came up with some games during the examination, such as giving the boy the stethoscope to listen to my heart. If I was using this dying boy for my education, I later wrote, "I had to give him *something* in return."

Once again, I struggled with my role. My resident had made me the official blood drawer for one of the boys. Although I was able to obtain the blood, he cringed and screamed whenever I came into the room, making it difficult for me to develop any type of relationship with him. His mother told me that he was starting kindergarten in the fall, but we both knew he would never finish school. Fortunately, many of the pediatric residents and attendings prided themselves on dealing with such profoundly challenging cases. The pediatricians' egos, I wrote, were smaller than those of other physicians. I learned a great deal from their ease at interacting with both the sick children and their parents.

One Saturday morning, I decided to visit one of my patients, a boy with cystic fibrosis whose parents had gone to New Jersey for the weekend. We had bonded earlier in the week, I wrote, because he was "manic," full of energy despite his debilitating illness. He had given me a gift of a painted clay pizza. But on Saturday, he was crying. We just sat and talked. My dad surely would have approved of this intervention: no fancy antibiotics, just words. Suddenly it mattered less that I could not always read the *New York Times*.

My next rotation was internal medicine. This was the big one. I enjoyed all my third-year rotations but had little doubt that I would pursue a career in some aspect of internal medicine, like my father. I was no surgeon, and my pediatrics rotation showed me that I did not have the strength to deal with sick children. Besides, medicine, which involved the care of patients with a huge range of fascinating illnesses, had a puzzle-solving aspect that I loved. As of the mid-1980s, the wards at Columbia still had resident labs, in which students and residents performed their own Gram stains, blood counts, and other tests and then used the results to guide their therapeutic decisions. Having grown up with my father, I believed that this type of hands-on medicine was the only way to be a doctor.

But the rotation at Columbia was not without its drama. On the first day, my very capable intern handed me the scut beeper, the pager used by nurses to reach the doctor assigned to cover a large number of patients in the private Harkness Pavilion. The fact that I was not a doctor mattered little to my intern, who saw this as a tremendous opportunity for me to learn how to draw blood, place intravenous lines, and evaluate patients—and spare himself busywork.

If I needed help, I was to page him on his personal beeper. The trouble was that I was in way over my head. I was not especially good at doing procedures and had almost no experience evaluating medical patients with chest pain, headaches, or low blood pressure.

Welcome to medical education circa 1984. In 1978, Stephen Bergman, using the pen name Samuel Shem, had published a book called *The House of God*, an autobiographical account of the experiences of a group of physicians doing their residencies in internal medicine at Boston's Beth Israel Hospital—the site of my father's training. My classmates and I had all read it. The book was often cynical, portraying residency as a sort of game that pitted the overworked, dedicated, and nearly all male residents against almost everyone else in the hospital: nurses, administrators, boneheaded senior physicians, and, most notably, patients. Among the terms that *The House of God* popularized was *GOMER*, which stood for "Get Out of My Emergency Room" and described a stereotypical elderly, demented nursing-home patient who supposedly had no business being admitted to an acute-care hospital. There were also a series of laws, which included "Gomers don't die" and "The only good admission is a dead admission."

I wish I remembered what I thought of the book when I first read it, probably as a first- or second-year medical student. Bergman, who became a psychiatrist, intended for his book to teach empathy by criticizing the dehumanizing process of training. I understand this now, but that is absolutely not how most of the Columbia house staff viewed *The House of God*. To them, it was more of a how-to manual for getting through residency. Patients, whether gomers or not, were the antagonists, making seemingly endless demands, not following orders, or deteriorating just as we were trying to go to sleep or go home. Our heroes were colleagues who could turf patients to other services. House officers praised as "walls" their fellow residents who sent potential admissions home from the emergency room. The degree to which life imitated art at Columbia was best demonstrated by the fact that one of our residents explicitly imitated the book's Fat Man, a legendary doctor who dispensed wisdom and sarcasm in equal doses.

It may sound as if I disdained this sort of behavior, but I did not. Medical students generally worship their residents and I was no exception. They were smart, efficient, funny, and—most important—supremely confident. We all wanted to be just like them. And the residents on several rotations worked over a hundred hours a week. Many of their on-call shifts lasted up to thirty-six hours with no opportunity for them to sleep. In such circumstances, who could begrudge them a little name-calling or self-congratulation when they managed to dump a patient onto another service or hospital?

Still, when I wasn't laughing, I was quite upset by some of these antics. I had been part of a small group of medical students who had gathered during our first year to read an excerpt from the book *Getting Rid of Patients* by Terry Mizrahi, a sociologist who had observed the behavior of overworked house officers and was utterly appalled. At what point did these methods for blowing off steam truly lead to disrespect for—and even inferior care of—sick patients?

The dynamic was much the same during my second five-week internal medicine stint at St. Luke's, a Columbia affiliate located fifty blocks south, with a few additional ethical issues thrown in. My very capable but busy intern offered me the opportunity to forge his name on orders that I wrote for the patients I was following. It reflected his confidence in my abilities, and, unfortunately, I agreed. In retrospect, I was lucky not to have made some type of egregious error. In another case, I was the only member of the team who argued that an alcoholic patient be given a pass to take care of some business and then return to the hospital. My colleagues all believed that it was a ploy for him to go and drink. My opinion, which did not carry the day, possibly reflected my great naivete. But I was also trying to put into practice some of what I had learned about the limits of paternalism. Was it really so terrible for a perennially sick patient to get a little break from the hospital, or were the doctors merely asserting their power? One of the highlights of my St. Luke's experience was caring for patients in Scrymser, the last open ward in New York City, a huge hall in which patients' beds, separated by curtains, were arranged in a semicircle around the nurses' station. It was like walking into medicine's past, which I of course loved.

I enjoyed the rest of the third-year rotations and my fourth-year electives. Direct patient care was enormously rewarding and made me want to read all about the diseases I encountered. One rotation that I unexpectedly enjoyed was surgery. I knew I was too clumsy to become a surgeon and did not have the traditional gung-ho mentality. But for someone interested in the history of medicine, the specialty was fertile. Surgeons had particular reverence for brethren who had taught them particular techniques or invented specific operations. So when I held clamps in the operating room, I was quizzed on legendary nineteenth-century surgeons such as Theodor Billroth, who pioneered partial stomach removal for ulcers, and Charles McBurney, who pinpointed the best place to make an incision when an inflamed appendix needed to be removed. I scrubbed in with the well-spoken patrician surgeon Philip Wiedel, who performed a similar type of meticulous mastectomy—in which every individual blood vessel was tied off—that the famous William Halsted himself had advocated. The operation took many hours but was a chapter in the history of medicine that would disappear within a decade as Wiedel's generation of surgeons retired.

I also greatly appreciated my rotation on neurology, in part because the long length of stays for patients with strokes allowed time for more meaningful interactions. In addition, the neurologists seemed to be the last physicians who viewed the proliferation of CT scans and other sophisticated diagnostic imaging as threatening to the intellectual nature of medicine. Several of the neurology attendings even forbade the students to give the results of head CT scans until after the team, revisiting the brain's anatomy and function, attempted to determine where the patient's lesion was likely to be. This was my father's medicine, pure and simple. The patient, as opposed to the disease, was front and center. But within a few years, as more and more X-rays and scans were routinely obtained in the emergency room prior to admission, most senior physicians—in neurology and other fields—simply allowed the answer to the case to be revealed. The traditional exercise of diagnosing challenging diseases, which required prolonged contact with patients and had fostered the careers of many great physicians, was becoming a dying art.

By this time, I had decided that I wanted to stay in New York City for my internal medicine residency—preferably at Columbia, where I had grown quite comfortable. During my fourth year, I was able to return to several of my outside interests, including helping to write the annual comedy show and serving as the musical director for the Bard Hall Players' production of *Pippin*. What my classmates and I were really waiting for, however, was Match Day, the day on which fourth-year medical students learn where they will be doing their residencies. Students list their preferred choices, and residency programs create lists of their preferred students. A computer does the rest. I had listed Columbia first, but it was far from clear that I would match there, in part due to my lackluster performance during the first two years of medical school. But my third- and fourth-year rotations had gone very well, and I had bonded with several attendings in the Department of Medicine. When I opened my envelope on Match Day, I received good news. Plus, many close medical school classmates would become my fellow interns and residents.

Although my dad had not dropped me off at medical school, he was surely not going to miss my graduation in May 1986, twenty-eight years after his own medical school graduation. In addition to him, my mother, my sister, and both grandmothers—Pearl and Jessie—attended. My father noted the absence of Mannie and Meyer with great regret. Regarding the two of us, he wrote in his journals that he was "drawing ever closer to me as a friend and colleague, not just as a son."

At this time, my father was abuzz not only with my graduation from medical school but with news of his recent humanitarian trip with his brother, Allan, to the Soviet Union, where they had met with a large number of "courageous and resolute" Jewish refuseniks, individuals prohibited from emigrating out of the country. The two brothers had brought with them forbidden reading materials, gifts, and emotional support for the cause. They had also helped a few refuseniks get permission to come to the United States for medical treatment. Like his year of sitting shivah for my grandfather, this was another one of my father's episodic, but highly intense, interactions with his faith. Throughout these years, my father had also remained engrossed with the Holocaust, reading Elie Wiesel and collecting stories from relatives, colleagues, and patients. Coincidentally, during an airport layover on their trip home, Phil and Allan had met and chatted with the famed Nazi hunter Simon Wiesenthal, who had devoted his life to avenging the deaths of his fellow Jews. My dad characterized helping the refuseniks as a way for him and his brother—who had avoided the Holocaust—to repay their "Jewish debt."

It was fitting that my father would invoke this sentiment as I was graduating from medical school, as it had been one of his prime reasons for becoming a doctor. Meanwhile, an award that I received at graduation spoke to my own motivations as a medical student—one who had tried to maintain a broad range of interests while becoming a physician. P&S awarded the annual Joseph Garrison Parker Prize to the graduate "who exemplifies through a continuation of his or her personal interest and activities in art, music, literature or the public interest, the fact that living and learning go together." I was pleased to receive the award even though I realized that it probably went to the most restless student.

I was, of course, determined to maintain my outside life despite the rigors of internship, which began at the end of June. One of my fellow interns, Eric Stevens, and I planned to go jogging together on mornings when neither of us was on call in the hospital. The jogging lasted for only a few weeks. I started the year with perhaps the two hardest rotations—first oncology and then the medical intensive care unit (MICU)—and things never really eased up. It was a year in which I learned to be a doctor, confronted more intriguing ethical issues, and, truth be told, struggled to keep my patients front and center.

The learning curve for an intern is incredibly steep. I had spent a lot of time on the wards as a medical student but always with close supervision. Not surprisingly, it was not until I had my own patients—and was their primary caretaker—that I developed the skills to practice medicine competently. My oncology patients were incredibly sick. Many of them had neutropenic sepsis, a common complication of chemotherapy in which a patient gets a blood infection because of a low white blood cell count. Others were bleeding, requiring continual transfusions of red blood cells and platelets.

Just as my father recalled specific patients who played seminal roles in his education, so, too, did I. During my first week of internship, I was called to see a previously stable patient with pancreatic cancer whose blood pressure had fallen. When I entered the room, his entire body was shaking. Although I had never seen this before, I knew immediately that he was having rigors, a sign of a bacterial infection in the blood. I later realized that as I was speaking to the patient, I had reflexively opened up his intravenous drip to full speed, something crucial for low blood pressure. It was one of those moments that built my confidence. I called my resident for help. We gave the patient antibiotics and transferred him to the intensive care unit.

The other thing I remember from this case was the patient's fear. He asked me if he was going to be all right. I had been a doctor for only a few days and I was already encountering an extraordinarily difficult question. I knew that the patient was going to die from his cancer. I was not sure if he would recover from the infection, but there was a good chance. So I focused on that issue and told him I believed the infection was treatable and he would be getting antibiotics momentarily. That the patient was Jewish, roughly my dad's age, and had a disease similar to my mother's only made the situation more emotionally charged. But at the same time, perhaps it helped the patient to be cared for by someone who could have been his son. I was getting a better sense of the sort of holistic interventions that my father made at the Mount Sinai.

On call nights, I cross-covered patients who did not have cancer. One of them was an elderly man who seemed to go into severe heart failure every fourth night, just when I was on call. Each time, he looked like he was about to die. The first two times I called the covering resident for help and we administered oxygen, diuretics, and other medications. But the third time I thought to myself, *I know how to do this*—and I did.

At times the decision to strut my stuff was not mine. On one call night in the middle of my internship, I received my fourth and fifth admissions just before midnight, which was the deadline for new cases. They were both incredibly sick; one had severe emphysema and the other a high fever, clouded mental status, and a recent history of heavy alcohol use. The covering resident, who I worked with only on call nights, admitted both cases with me and then announced he was going to sleep.

"But we have to do a spinal tap on the alcoholic," I reminded him.

"No, *you* have to do it," he replied.

"But he's agitated," I said. "How can I do it by myself?"

"Tie him down with a sheet and have the nurse help you."

And then he left.

It was one of those *House of God* moments. I knew that I could not complain or I'd be considered a weenie by him and some of my other colleagues. So I did what I had to do with the help of a very sympathetic and capable nurse. Fortunately, the patient did fine. Even better, my regular resident laid into the admitting resident the following morning for having given me two such hard cases so late at night.

But the place that my colleagues and I really learned medicine was in the medical intensive care unit, both during my first rotation early in internship and several subsequent stints there over the next two years. The patients were incredibly sick with multiple failing organ systems. In managing all of these simultaneous problems, we really learned how the body worked. For example, patients could have far too much fluid in their bodies but not enough in their blood vessels. Low blood pressure required completely different treatment depending on whether it was caused by heart failure or a blood infection. Blood transfusions were the best way to hydrate a patient; sugar water the worst.

All the unit's attending physicians were excellent, but MICU director Glenda Garvey—whom I had befriended as a student—was, by far, the most memorable. The daughter of two physicians and the granddaughter of another, she had been an English and American literature major at Wellesley College before matriculating at P&S and had stayed on for her residency in internal medicine. There were a smattering of senior women physicians at Columbia, but none quite like Garvey. Despite her gender, Garvey practiced medicine in a manner that was reminiscent of legendary male internists like Paul Beeson, Robert Loeb, and Louis Weinstein. Her knowledge, in her specialty of infectious diseases and in other areas, was immense. Rounds with Garvey were methodical and lengthy, but that was because she insisted on learning every physical finding and laboratory value. "Knowing your stuff," one of her trainees noted, "was the highest priority." I suspect that residents who rounded with Garvey in the MICU all had some type of eureka moment in which they suddenly felt confident in caring for the sickest patients imaginable. Such knowledge was fundamental to becoming a great doctor—no matter how committed one was to patient-centered care. As a woman practicing top-notch intensive care medicine at a prestigious medical center, Garvey was a particularly impressive role model for my female colleagues. Her own male medical school classmates had been so perplexed by the presence of a small number of women that they had once sent them all roses on Valentine's Day. But now Garvey was no longer a curiosity. As one P&S student wrote years later in a blog post, "Dr. Garvey is cool, Dr. Garvey is funny. Dr. Garvey is trim, chic, well-dressed, and looks coolly elegant in a fur coat . . . Dr. Garvey is really, *really* smart. She knows everything. *Everything*, dammit. But unlike many doctors who teach us, she never makes you feel stupid just because you don't happen to know everything yet. Because she's chill like that, yo."

Garvey's joy when patients improved was palpable. Without any embarrassment, she would proclaim urine made by recovering kidneys "golden goodness." She insisted that the junior resident on call in the MICU phone her late at night to touch base on the patients. When it was my turn to do so, I felt like one of the residents or fellows my father spoke with during our family vacations. "Now," Garvey once said to me when she and I finished one of these conversations, "I can go to sleep."

What was discussed less in the unit, however, was how a patient's prognosis should affect medical decisions; even patients who did not seem likely to pull through were treated aggressively. Perhaps because her approach to medicine was so old school, Garvey immersed herself in the medical details of patients rather than scrutinizing the possible ethical ramifications of our interventions. Typical was the very first patient we rounded on in late July of my internship. He was an intravenous drug user in his forties who had been on a ventilator for many weeks with failure of multiple organs. He had just about every tube possible stuck into his body and was massively swollen and unresponsive. There were several other similar patients in the fourteen-bed ward.

To be sure, I was no expert in clinical medicine, let alone intensive care medicine. Nevertheless, having learned about the debates over end-of-life care in the Society and Medicine course, I was surprised to observe Garvey's daily focus on treating the patient's infections, fluid balance, and breathing status, seemingly without her paying any attention to whether such interventions were actually going to help the patient to recover. Other residents noticed this seeming imbalance as well.

Part of the problem was that, while medical schools like P&S were beginning to teach bioethics, there was nothing remotely close to an ethics or professionalism curriculum in most residency training programs—and Columbia's was no exception. Interestingly, however, there was a particularly enlightened pair of eyes and ears present in the MICU: Robert Zussman, a sociologist working with the Center for the Study of Society and Medicine who was doing fieldwork for a book on the ethics of intensive care medicine. Zussman, who wore a herringbone sports jacket in the MICU, symbolized what David Rothman had termed a "stranger at the bedside," a nonphysician who had come to exert a growing influence over medical decision making. Garvey had given Zussman permission to attend MICU rounds, but he made her uncomfortable, which we knew from how she raised her eyebrows when he offered an opinion. In *Intensive Care*, Zussman ultimately concluded that "moral education" in the unit was "hit or miss," as opposed to systematic. And he believed that the Columbia-Presbyterian MICU (called Outerboro in the book) was particularly "insistent" on "pursuing every therapeutic possibility, even for patients in apparently terminal stages of illness."

What was going on here? It is not surprising that practice lagged behind theory. It was easy to talk about the medical profession's ethical blind spots in the classroom but much harder to effect change on the wards. At the same time, patient care in the MICU exemplified the style of medicine that doctors of Garvey's generation had learned and with which they were comfortable: one where physicians made the tough decisions for patients. The increasingly important concept of informed consent, in which patients and families made educated choices using information provided by doctors, played only a small role at Columbia, Zussman found. During the course of his research in the MICU, only eight patients declined a procedure, and seven of the eight either changed their minds or were overruled. Paternalism still ruled the day. Until the attending physicians said otherwise, the treatment of my first MICU patient that July would remain a full-court press.

I had encountered a similar mind-set during my previous month on the oncology service. Many of the patients who were deteriorating did not seem to know that they had terminal cancer. Thus, when the house staff raised questions with them about how aggressive their care should be and whether a transfer to the MICU would be appropriate, patients were often confused or even angry. Whereas some of these patients probably knew their prognoses and were in denial, it was clear that some of the senior Columbia oncologists were purposely avoiding these types of discussions, something that the social scientist Nicholas A. Christakis would later confirm in a series of studies on doctor-patient communication at the end of life. When I began to study bioethics and the history of medicine formally in succeeding years, I would learn why autonomy and other patient-centered strategies had become so crucial and why so many physicians continued to resist them. One of those physicians was my father.

Although I tried to incorporate bioethical teachings into the care of my patients, it was not easy. In addition to our relative inexperience on the wards, my colleagues and I were always exhausted. If we had a choice between raising ethical concerns and going home to sleep, we almost always found the latter more appealing. Fatigue remained a particular problem for me, given my inability to grab an hour of sleep whenever the opportunity arose. Overnight call on the wards was only one out of every four nights, but there was not yet a night-float system, in which doctors covered patients at night in order to ease the burden of the daytime staff. As a result, I was generally up all night dealing with my own patients and those I was covering. That meant that every four days, I worked a thirty-six-hour shift, from roughly 7 a.m. to 7 p.m. the following day. I had not previously been much of a coffee drinker, but that changed. By the afternoon I was post-call, I simply poured it down the hatch in order to stay awake and—frankly—try not to kill someone due to my exhaustion.

Twenty years later, for my book on famous patients, I wrote about the well-known Libby Zion case, in which an eighteen-year-old girl died at New York Hospital in 1984. Zion, who had been admitted for fever and agitation, underwent an abrupt deterioration for unclear reasons and died within twelve hours of her arrival at the hospital. As was the custom at the time, the physicians who admitted Zion were house officers covering dozens of patients and working two-day shifts. I interviewed her father, Sidney Zion, a journalist and former prosecutor who, in the wake of Libby's death, had successfully carried out a passionate and often harsh crusade to force the medical establishment to implement shorter resident work hours and better attending-level supervision. There were some physicians who objected to the night-float shifts that Zion and other reformers advocated, arguing that doctors in training could achieve mastery of diseases only by watching patients for the first two days of their admissions, but I did not share that view. What we were doing was crazy.

Ultimately, it was exhaustion and time pressure that jeopardized the one thing that had made so many of us go into medicine: patient care. Reflecting on medicine in the postwar years, when the average hospitalized patient was much less sick, Paul Beeson recalled having lots of time: "Time to talk and time to think about our patients." Yet—just as detailed in Shem's and Mizrahi's books—I often had to choose between having some free time and doing the best for my patients. Disturbingly, I found myself behaving in ways that I had never thought I would, even occasionally seeing patients as my enemies. One particular case underscored for me how foolish this sort of attitude was.

I was on call. It was about 5:30 a.m. and I had finally finished admitting my patients and doing all the cross coverage. I was in the call room and hoped I could get about ninety minutes of sleep before morning rounds. I was utterly exhausted. I got into the bed and actually fell asleep. Ten minutes later, my beeper went off. It was a nurse calling to report that one of the patients I was covering for another intern was having chest pain. I asked if anyone had done an electrocardiogram (EKG) or gotten vital signs, knowing full well that the answer was likely to be no. "How does the patient look?" I asked. "Okay," she said, "but I don't know him very well."

I looked at the sign-out form I had been given. The patient was a middle-aged Dominican man in his fifties who had been admitted for chest pain but was supposed to go home the following day. The form said that he was on Tylenol for pain. I so wanted to go back to sleep. Couldn't I just tell the nurse to give him some Tylenol and then go see him at 7 a.m.?

Well, no. I would not have been able to sleep anyway. But I was mad. Mad at the system and mad at the patient for waking me up. When I walked into the patient's room, however, I must have either said or thought, "Holy shit!" He was sitting bolt upright in bed, breathing forty times a minute, which is an extremely high respiratory rate. A quick examination revealed him to be in flash pulmonary edema: his lungs had filled with fluid. I did what I had to do: I started oxygen, put in an intravenous line, gave him a diuretic by vein, and placed a nitroglycerin pill under his tongue. I also asked the nurses to page the anesthesiologist on call to intubate the patient and put him on a ventilator.

Less than an hour later, things had become much quieter on the ward. The patient had been successfully transferred to the cardiac intensive care unit (CCU). I reminded myself that I had genuinely considered going back to sleep instead of seeing the patient. The patient was lucky, but so was I. By this time, it was nearing 7:00. There was no point in going back to the call room. I just went and got my coffee.

Months later, a man animatedly ran up to me and hugged me. I did not recognize him. "Doctor, Doctor, you saved my life," he said in broken English. I immediately knew who he was then. Fortunately, he did not know the whole story!

Perhaps the most disturbing event of my internship happened late one Friday afternoon when I was called about another patient with chest pain. I was busy dealing with a different problem, so I sent my medical student to do an electrocardiogram on the patient. I arrived a few minutes later and when I saw the tracing, I'm not sure what looked worse: the patient, who was pale, sweating, and had a very low blood pressure, or the EKG, which had the classic tombstone pattern consistent with an acute heart attack. My student did not look so good either. There were a million things to do, including putting in additional intravenous lines, giving the patient fluid, and getting him to the CCU as soon as possible. I needed help. The medical student, who was quite good, was nearly useless in this emergency, so I had him page my immediate supervisor, a junior resident. But the resident did not answer his beeper. In desperation, I told the student to go to the nurses' station and ask any doctors there to come and help us. There was only one present: a popular, competent attending cardiologist. The student practically begged him to come, but the attending said no and told him to call his resident. Out of options, I did what I had to do: I called a code, thereby alerting the on-call anesthesiologist and the rest of the medical staff that there was an emergency. Such codes are normally limited to cardiac arrests, when patients' hearts have actually stopped. My patient was still breathing and had a blood pressure, but I felt that I had no choice. Finally, the help I needed arrived and we transferred the patient to intensive care.

The attending's refusal to help us, however, always stuck with me. I am certain he was truly busy and perhaps even late to other patient-related commitments. But what kind of physician would not have pitched in to save a possibly dying patient until help arrived? Of course, this doctor is hardly the only one who has acted this way. My wife tells the story of a physician whose children she babysat when she was a teenager. One night, as he was driving her home, they approached a car crash. Rather than stopping to assist, this physician drove back to his house and switched to the car that did not have MD on its license plate.

It was hard not to think about my father—who I could not imagine ignoring a human in distress—when reflecting on these episodes. Once, when I was a teenager, he had pulled a child out of the back seat of a terribly mangled car that had crashed near our house. The child's mother, who was driving, did not survive, but the girl did. And somehow, my father had always managed, despite a busy consultation service, teaching responsibilities, and clinical research, to keep his primary focus on doing what was best for his patients. Whether I felt burned out or not, the right choice was clear to me.

Another reason I often thought about my dad during my internship and residency was the abrupt appearance of tuberculosis and AIDS. Tuberculosis, which had been the leading cause of death in New York and other cities in the early 1900s, had never actually gone away; it quietly persisted among disadvantaged urban populations. Now it was back with a vengeance, thanks to cutbacks in public health funding, the rise of homelessness in the 1980s, and, it would turn out, the immunosuppression caused by AIDS.

I wish I could say otherwise, but the wise physicians of Columbia (and many other medical centers) were ill prepared for the return of what was once known as the great white plague. Some attending physicians, not having seen a case of the disease in decades, forgot how communicable it could be. On rounds one morning during internship, my attending brought us into the room of a patient with active tuberculosis to excitedly demonstrate the succussion splash, a finding first described by the ancient Greek physician Hippocrates: a characteristic noise heard when one shook a patient who had a large lung cavity containing both air and fluid. The patient coughed the entire time. The masks we wore were woefully inadequate to prevent the transmission of tuberculosis. Indeed, within a few months, my tuberculosis skin test had turned positive, indicating that I had become infected with the bacteria (although not ill from it). Many of my fellow residents also became infected during our three-year tenure. It was not only the medical profession that missed the boat. New York City health officials took far too long to realize that the city's burgeoning homeless shelters, including an enormous one located across the street from Columbia-Presbyterian, were breeding grounds for tuberculosis, including the drug-resistant types.

We were also insufficiently careful regarding AIDS, which was caused by a virus, eventually called the human immunodeficiency virus (HIV), and led to a series of common and uncommon infections. As my onetime Columbia colleagues Ronald Bayer and Gerald M. Oppenheimer later documented in their excellent book *AIDS Doctors*, physicians across the country—even infectious diseases specialists—downplayed the potential infectivity of the HIV virus. During my pediatrics rotation, one of my fellow medical students drew blood each morning on the hospital's first AIDS baby without wearing gloves. I remember seeing blood on his hands. It seemed sort of crazy to me, but none of the physicians rebuked him. Interestingly, however, the message that we should protect the privacy of AIDS patients came through loud and clear. Whether due to fears of causing panic among other patients or a sincere effort to prevent AIDS patients from losing their jobs or their health insurance or both, there was an informal edict that we should not actually write *AIDS* or *HIV* in the medical charts. Such efforts, while well-meaning, led us to write some pretty convoluted notes that probably did not enhance the care of our AIDS population.

It was particularly interesting for me that just as I was beginning my medical career, infectious diseases were dominating the wards and the headlines. Doctors like my father and Louis Weinstein, who for years had been preaching about the misuse of antimicrobials and the development of drug-resistant bacteria, would have been the first to say that serious infections had not gone away. But the control of infectious diseases such as polio, rheumatic fever, and diphtheria had indisputably been a public health triumph. Now, once again, infectious diseases specialists were taking care of the sickest patients in the hospital. In the case of AIDS, young previously healthy people, mostly gay men at first, were being admitted with severe infections that often killed them in a few days. Many of these were the rare so-called opportunistic infections seen only in individuals with severely depressed immune systems. I vividly remember admitting to the MICU a man in his late twenties who was a weight lifter and had been in terrific shape. But pneumocystis pneumonia (PCP) had entirely eaten away his lungs; he died almost immediately. It took all the expertise of Glenda Garvey, Harold Neu, and their infectious diseases colleagues at Columbia and across the country to juggle antimicrobial agents and buy time for these unfortunate AIDS victims.

As the head of the MICU, Garvey probably saw most of these patients before they died. Over time, there were fewer gay men and many more homeless people with histories of psychiatric problems and intravenous drug use. The notion that these patients somehow deserved to get AIDS due to their aberrant lifestyles was rampant in the media. Some of my coworkers on the wards of our hospital, I must confess, felt the same.

But Garvey would have none of this. Although she rivaled any of her colleagues in her knowledge of medicine, Garvey was profoundly affected by these dying souls. Was it because she was a senior woman physician in a hospital that had too few others? Perhaps. We residents were overtired and often cynical, but we took notice and hoped that we would one day care as much. As one of Garvey's students, Steve Miller, later wrote, "I saw her holding the hands of dying AIDS patients, in comas, when most others were afraid to touch them."

Well after several Columbia colleagues and I had finished our training, we continued to organize periodic reunion dinners with Garvey. Unfortunately, she developed colon cancer in the late 1990s and eventually died of it in 2004 at the age of sixty-one. I'd like to think that Garvey, who had no children of her own, saw this group of mentees—trained by her to provide consummate care to their patients—as her surrogate kids. After her death, Columbia wisely began a teaching academy in her name.

If tuberculosis and AIDS represented enormous challenges even for experienced clinicians, the two diseases provided a boon for medical historians and bioethicists, who were called upon to revisit past epidemic infectious diseases and discuss such tricky issues as quarantining the sick. In fact, tuberculosis would become the main focus of my own research once I became a fellow and graduate student.

CHAPTER FIVE

Forging My Own Path

Students and house officers interested in careers in bioethics, medical history, or the medical humanities often ask me how I became an MD-PhD. I tell them it was mostly good luck and good timing. Just as my father had taken advantage of an opening in Louis Weinstein's infectious diseases fellowship program, I applied to the Robert Wood Johnson Foundation's Clinical Scholars Program at a time when it was supporting researchers interested in history and bioethics.

I had been exposed to these fields as a medical student and resident, but as a Clinical Scholar at the University of Washington in Seattle, I began formal study and met leading researchers. I had not particularly planned to focus my research on the years after World War II, but exploring the transition from medical paternalism to patient autonomy made a lot of sense for someone interested in the history of medicine and bioethics. The postwar era was when the ground began to shake under the comfortable model of physician-dominated medical practice that had existed for centuries. My research into the triumph of autonomy meant that I would also explore a series of ethical issues—including human experimentation, conflict of interest, and truth-telling—that directly called into question the behaviors of my father and his generation of physicians. Our competing perspectives led to spirited arguments and, at times, genuine tension between us. The world of medicine had split apart over the previous twenty years and my dad and I seemed to be on opposite sides.

I never heard of the Clinical Scholars Program during my days as a house officer. The Department of Medicine at Columbia was a very traditional place and the vast majority of residents subspecialized in fields like cardiology, gastrointestinal diseases, and infectious diseases. Only rarely did a graduate choose to go into general internal medicine, even though all the residents maintained a general medicine clinic throughout their three years in the program. I knew that I did not want to subspecialize, but I had no idea what I wanted to do. Like several of my other indecisive peers, I began a stint as an attending physician in Columbia-Presbyterian's emergency department, actually earning a reasonable salary for the first time.

When I learned about the Robert Wood Johnson program, I was immediately intrigued. Clinical Scholars spent two years at one of six sites across the country, learning research skills, being mentored, and usually earning advanced degrees. Most of the scholars, I would learn, were studying epidemiology or health services research, but several others were interested in history or bioethics.

But any decision to apply to the Clinical Scholars Program was complicated by the fact that on Christmas Day of 1989, I had become engaged to Cathy Seibel, a federal prosecutor in the Southern District of New York. To say that Cathy had no interest in leaving New York—even for two years—is a major understatement. She had been born and raised in the area, gone to Fordham Law School, clerked for a federal judge in Brooklyn, and landed the job of her dreams in Manhattan. Two of the Clinical Scholars sites that fit my interests were located relatively nearby, one at the University of Pennsylvania and one at Yale University. These programs raised the possibility that Cathy could keep her job and one or both of us would take on a longer commute. But another logical location for me was the University of Washington in Seattle. The ultimate choice of location was made by the program.

I eventually listed all three universities as places that I would be willing to attend, and Cathy extracted a promise from me that if we had to leave New York for two years, she could pick where we lived for the rest of our lives. When the Clinical Scholars Program called me with their decision, it turned out to be Seattle. Although the city was regularly listed as one of the most livable in America, and our friends and family foresaw a great adventure for two inveterate New Yorkers, Cathy was not happy, except for me. But it helped that she was able to find a position in the US Attorney's Office in Seattle. We also doubled the size of our New York City apartment while paying only half our old rent.

Once I arrived in Seattle in July 1991, I knew the opportunity would be a spectacular one for me. My father agreed, even though he originally wished that I had chosen a career in a cutting-edge field like immunology or geographic medicine. He predicted that my fellowship would be an "important milestone" in my life, just as his training in infectious diseases had been for him. My fellow clinical scholars, both in Seattle and across the country, were incredibly bright and motivated. The directors of the University of Washington program, Thomas Inui, Thomas Koepsell, and Richard Deyo, were terrific mentors. And the medical school's Department of Medical History and Ethics was populated with top-notch faculty, including chairman Albert R. Jonsen. A former Jesuit priest, Jonsen was one of the founding fathers of the field of bioethics, having sat on the influential National Commission for the Protection of Human Subjects of Biomedical and Behavioral Research and the President's Commission on the Study of Ethical Problems in Medicine. I formally enrolled in the department's master's program, which I planned to complete by June 1992.

In addition to doing my coursework, I served as a research assistant for Jonsen, who was writing a history of the bioethics movement, *The Birth of Bioethics*. This task was well suited to my interest in history: researching how physicians had addressed ethical issues in medicine before the rise of the bioethics during the 1970s and 1980s. Working directly with Jonsen was a great advantage for another reason. To some extent, Jonsen's book was a response to David

Rothman's book on the rise of bioethics, *Strangers at the Bedside*, which he had researched during my years as a medical student and resident at Columbia and published in 1991. The two books, both excellent, told the same story in dramatically different ways. Rothman, the historian, situated the bioethics movement firmly among the social movements of the 1960s and 1970s that had rejected traditionally powerful organizations. Jonsen, in contrast, had written more of a disciplinary history that examined the careers of the theologians, philosophers, and other academics who—like him—became the first leaders of the bioethics movement. For a young historian, it was a lesson in historiography (the history of telling history) that I would never forget and would use in my own research and teaching.

Despite their distinctive approaches, both Rothman and Jonsen stressed a common theme: prior to the era of bioethics, physicians had often overstepped their power and, at times, treated patients as somehow less than human. Meanwhile, both authors applauded the role of bioethics in asking what had gone wrong with the moral bearings of the medical profession.

There was great variability in the nascent field of bioethics, not only in the disciplinary background of its membership but also in their assessment of what behaviors should be labeled objectionable or unethical. For example, though the historian Rothman and the theologian Jonsen both liberally criticized the actions of many specific physicians, neither were doctor bashers. In contrast, Yale University psychiatrist Jay Katz more directly laid blame on his fellow physicians for deliberately excluding patients from active participation in their care. Doctors, he wrote, had created a "silent world of doctor and patient," in which they wrote orders that patients were supposed to follow and never question. These negative assessments of the medical profession mirrored the contemporaneous work of critics such as Michel Foucault and Ivan Illich, who had no formal connection with the field of bioethics.

At times, this scholarship made me feel defensive. Although I had been a physician for only five years, I had enough admiration for my peers and superiors to worry that bioethicists tended to tar the medical profession with too broad a brush. Issues that seemed black-and-white around a conference table—such as whether to let a human "vegetable" die or tell a cancer patient every last bit of information about his or her condition—were considerably more complicated when one was dealing with actual patients and families.

Nevertheless, I was far too immersed in the worlds of history and bioethics not to embrace the basic core of what these scholars and critics were arguing: Physicians, while perhaps having noble motives, often behaved in ways that could be described only as patronizing, paternalistic, and uncaring. They routinely misled patients, disregarded ethical codes designed to protect the rights of experimental subjects, and failed to take informed consent seriously. Moreover, I had become a full-fledged fan of efforts designed to rectify this situation: the passage of do-not-resuscitate laws that empowered patients and families to select or decline cardiopulmonary resuscitation; the call for physicians and hospitals to tell the truth when a medical error occurred; and, most important, the insistence that there be true informed consent when a subject agreed to enter an experimental protocol or when a patient—such as a woman with breast cancer—agreed to a particular treatment.

This mind-set surely informed my choice of a dissertation topic. I had successfully completed my master's degree in medical history and ethics by June of 1992 and, with one year left in my Robert Wood Johnson fellowship, had decided to enter the PhD program in the University of Washington's Department of History. The plan was to take required courses for two semesters and then complete pre-dissertation exams in four subjects: the history of medicine, bioethics, the history of science, and twentieth-century US history. I would then look for a job, presumably in New York, and complete my dissertation long distance. I had been reading extensively in all these areas since my arrival in Seattle and in a few history courses I had taken at Columbia prior to the move. My ability to complete so much in two years reflected not only my hard work but also a supportive wife and a series of colleagues and mentors, including my dissertation advisor, James C. Whorton, who went out of their way to design a strategy for a practicing physician to become a legitimate PhD historian.

Several people suggested possible dissertation topics, such as a history of University of Washington physician Belding Scribner's arteriovenous shunt, which had made chronic kidney hemodialysis possible and led to the 1962 God Squad controversy that I had learned about during medical school. But what really interested me were some informal remarks I had heard about the treatment of tuberculosis in Seattle in the years after World War II. The physicians who staffed the city's Firland Sanatorium had apparently been the country's most aggressive advocates of forcible detention for tuberculosis patients who did not reliably take their medications. If these rumors were true, this topic, which seemed to demonstrate another possible example of the medical profession's excesses, would be an ideal way for me to combine my interests (and growing expertise) in history and ethics.

Of course, I needed to verify the story before embarking on such a major project. Fishing around one day in the University of Washington archives, I struck gold. In the papers of the Washington State chapter of the American Civil Liberties Union, I found letters written by Firland patients charging that "people who have had negative sputum for months may be placed under quarantine," that patients who drank beer while on approved leaves had a "very good chance of being thrown in jail," and that doctors—not judges—"may sentence a patient from one day to six months" on a locked ward within the sanatorium. These documents proved to be only the tip of the iceberg. I eventually got access to the actual Firland patient charts that contained not only many similar letters but proof of what the patients had charged. Firland's locked ward, officially established to detain actively infectious patients who represented public health threats, had become, in the words of one patient, "a jail in every sense of the word." Unfortunately, despite efforts to engage local ACLU representatives, little changed at Firland until the institution was closed in 1973.

What had made the Seattle doctors behave in this manner? It turned out that at the time, the city was home to a large population of itinerant workers, many of whom were poor alcoholics living in Seattle's Skid Road area. Confronted with a challenging population of patients who broke sanatorium rules, the physicians took it upon themselves to become policemen. This medical authority manifested itself in another, even less probable, manner. Firland surgeons removed portions of Skid Road alcoholics' lungs—even when such patients had inactive tuberculosis—on the assumption that the patients would revert to alcohol abuse upon release, fail to take their medications, and again develop active tuberculosis. The Firland staff unabashedly wrote in such patients' charts that they were ordering surgery for "sociological," as opposed to medical, reasons. A patient who was "Indian, alcoholic, a schoolteacher, and divorced," a former Firland surgeon told me, was "sure to get a resection." Even though partial lung removal most likely left enough lung tissue in place for the patient to live a normal life, surgery left scars and was not without risks. Moreover, it is almost impossible to imagine that these Skid Road patients were able to question the need for such operations.

My dissertation was completed in 1996 and eventually became my first book, *Contagion and Confinement*, published in 1998, after I had returned to Columbia as an assistant professor. My second book, *The Breast Cancer Wars*, contained even more dramatic examples of hubris from this era. Surgeons, often more impressed with their ability to perform heroic operations than with the actual value of such procedures, removed ribs, arms, and legs of certain patients with advanced cancers in an effort to remove every last cancer cell. "The purpose of the surgeon to divorce his patient from the cancer," coldly wrote George T. Pack in 1951, "appears to be limited solely by the ability of the human remnant to survive." One surgeon termed patient-activist Rose Kushner's pathbreaking 1975 book on breast cancer "a piece of garbage." Avoiding a radical mastectomy due to "feminine whims," another surgeon wrote derisively, would result in a "dead woman with a somewhat more pleasant-appearing chest wall."

I don't exactly recall when I started making connections between these types of statements and my father, but it was most likely in the early 1990s as I was pursuing my degrees in bioethics and history. To be sure, he had never had the occasion to lock up tuberculosis patients or to remove any organs, let alone limbs. But as I became more and more involved in studying the history of bioethics, I found worrisome parallels. One of the first I learned about was my father's participation in human experimentation in which informed consent had not been obtained from the subjects. We had been discussing such research in 1994 after the journalist Eileen Welsome broke the astounding story that the US government had funded hundreds of radiation experiments performed on unknowing Americans during the Cold War years.

"I did some similar experiments when I was an infectious diseases fellow," my father told me during a visit to Cleveland. The remark caught me by surprise. "Are you serious?" I recall exclaiming. He went on to explain that one of Louis Weinstein's many projects had involved determining blood levels of antimicrobial drugs after subjects received injections of the medication. Such research helped doctors figure out the best dosing schedules. Weinstein's team had conducted the experiments at the Wrentham State School, an institution for mentally disabled children, injecting the children despite the fact that they were not sick. The consent process, my father suspected, had been minimal. I immediately peppered him with questions. What did he think, in retrospect, about his participation?

"We did things you could never do now," he told me. Protocols, he believed, had changed for the better.

I asked my father whether he or any of his colleagues had raised eyebrows at the time of the experiments. Did anyone ever mention the post–World War II Nuremberg Code that specifically prohibited this type of research? The answer was an emphatic no.

"These institutions were glad to participate in prestigious research," my dad said. "And so were Weinstein's fellows."

When I looked up the Wrentham State School, which was located in Wrentham, Massachusetts, thirty miles south of Boston, it sounded eerily like the other institutions that populated articles and books that criticized unethical human experimentation. Wrentham, founded in 1906, housed what were originally called feebleminded and later mentally retarded children. It turns out that some of the radiation experiments unearthed by Welsome had taken place there in 1961, concurrently with the Weinstein group's investigation of antimicrobial-drug blood levels.

I knew from my own research that only a small minority of doctors from this era had raised objections or declined to participate in research on captive populations. For instance, two of them had refused to inject cancer cells into the elderly patients at Brooklyn's Jewish Chronic Disease Hospital and had even made their concerns known to the press. But my father had gone along. My initial outrage gradually turned to mild disappointment. I reasoned that my dad was not a very political person and had surely been focused on doing good science. Plus, compared to some of the other egregious ethical violations taking place, injection of probably harmless antimicrobials was less terrible. And other revered physicians had participated in similar experiments. Paul Beeson, for example, had performed X-rays and invasive catheterizations on patients without obtaining consent.

Yet one of the reasons my father and his peers participated in such research raised another ethical concern. Funding for much of the work done in Weinstein's laboratory came from the drug giant Eli Lilly, based in Indianapolis, Indiana. Lilly, a major manufacturer of antibiotics, was glad to fund research into the efficacy of their drugs performed by well-known and highly respected investigators like Louis Weinstein.

My father maintained close ties with Lilly once he moved to Cleveland. He often brought home interesting gifts that he received from Lilly's and other drug companies' representatives—often attractive women—given to him in exchange for his listening to information about their newest antibiotics. Although my dad prided himself on not prescribing new, expensive medications when earlier versions would do the trick, bioethicists would eventually conclude that such interactions represented a conflict of interest. More disturbing was the fact that Lilly had provided him with somewhere between five thousand and ten thousand dollars for a 1983 trip to China in exchange for his mentioning Lilly antibiotics in all his lectures. This type of arrangement would come under exceedingly close scrutiny by the late 1990s, especially when data revealed that such arrangements influenced doctors' prescribing practices even when they claimed they remained objective.

Speaking of conflict of interest, I confronted another questionable activity of my father's: his decision to serve as the actual or de facto doctor for a number of our family members. This issue was not a traditional topic in bioethics, but it raised important questions about the proper boundaries of the doctor-patient relationship. The American Medical Association was concerned enough to write in its 1993 Medical Code of Ethics that "physicians generally should not treat themselves or members of their immediate families." Among the objections raised were that doctors who cared for relatives could not be objective and that such patients would feel too intimidated to ever reject the advice of their in-family physician. "Because a clinical encounter with a family member is not a typical doctor-patient relationship," a 1999 ethics case study advised, "physicians caring for family members may tend to ignore standard guidelines, such as respecting a patient's right to decide about treatment, informing the patient about the risks and benefits of treatment and plausible alternatives, telling patients the truth and respecting confidentiality."

At some point, I asked my father about the illness and death of my maternal grandfather, Mannie, in 1975. I vaguely remembered him saying before Mannie died that he should not be dialyzed for his kidney failure, and now, as a practicing physician, I wanted more details. My dad reminded me that Mannie had experienced a series of small strokes, which was probably the reason for his mental deterioration. Mannie had been admitted to the hospital for abdominal pain and a surgeon had made the presumptive diagnosis of dead intestine. The only treatment would have been emergency surgery in an attempt to remove the affected tissue, and my grandfather's surviving that surgery was surely a long shot, given his age and concurrent illnesses. Hemodialysis to treat my grandfather's failing kidneys was also possible but did not make much sense unless his intestinal problem was fixed.

When I inquired further about the decision to forgo surgery and dialysis and instead make Mannie comfortable, it seemed clear that my father had made the choice by himself. Given the poor overall prognosis and his expertise, it was certainly a reasonable option. And doctors made many such unilateral decisions in the 1970s. But as someone studying bioethics, I felt uneasy with both my father's paternalism and his conflict of interest as the son-in-law of the patient. These concerns were validated years later when I read about Mannie's death in a series of journal entries. "The only thing I can say," my dad wrote in September 1975, "is that he was failing very quickly and this had to be the best way for him and for Nana [my grandmother Jessie]." Mannie, he added, had been "so very uncomfortable the last year of his life."

Was it possible that Mannie's quality of life, while unacceptable to my father, was actually tolerable from Mannie's perspective? To the best of my recollection, he was still very interactive and mobile, with a healthy appetite. Maybe Jessie, his primary caretaker, actually had an idea of what Mannie would have wanted in such a situation. Even if not, what if she was not yet ready to let go? And did my mother, his daughter, have any say in the matter? The journals contain no mention of my dad discussing options with Mannie, Jessie, or my mom.

Ten years later, he was at it again. In June 1986, his aunt Libba, who lived in a nursing home, was hospitalized at the Mount Sinai with cancer. He made the decision that surgery and other aggressive therapy would be inappropriate. In this instance, my father was not simply giving advice to other doctors; he was the actual attending physician in charge of her care. It was a true conflict of interest. The bind he had gotten himself into was clear from a contemporaneous journal entry: "I'm trying not to prolong her life," he wrote, "but it is difficult to do so." Elsewhere, he wrote: "Have Aunt Libba in the hospital, trying to perform 'passive euthanasia.'" The house staff actually objected to his "minimalist approach" to his aunt's treatment.

Fast-forward to 1993. I can't recall if my father and I discussed his cousin Donald, who was dying from prostate cancer at that time. But his journal entries again revealed his inclination to influence the care of his dying relatives, even if it meant inserting himself into discussions between his family members and their physicians. In this case, my dad worried that Donald's pain and suffering were not being adequately treated.

It might be argued that in these cases, my father was merely serving as an intermediary, helping his relatives ensure that their loved ones received competent medical care that was both personal and efficient. But his concerns about the appropriateness of certain interventions—most notably the use of antibiotics and CPR, feeding tubes and intensive care—went far beyond offering logistical solutions. Rather, my father believed that many well-meaning physicians and hospitals had lost sight of the basic human gesture of allowing a person to die in peace, free from suffering. It was his job, he thought, to encourage—even insist—that they do so.

It might not seem logical, at first glance, to expect an infectious diseases consultant to become such a fierce advocate of the concept that came to be called medical futility. After all, physicians generally called in infectious-disease experts to cure infections and help patients recover. Early in his career, my dad saw this as his role. "When I was younger, it was easier to treat sick people," he later reflected. "If they survived the infection I was called to manage, fine. If not, I didn't give it a second thought, since I'd done *my* best and other factors . . . were responsible for the outcome."

But over time, things changed. In the hospital setting, my father was often called to consult on extremely sick patients, many of whom had spent weeks or months there, had acquired especially complicated infections, and had little or no chance of recovery. Some of these individuals had long since ceased to live at home but bounced back and forth between nursing homes and the hospital. The problem, my father believed, was that too many of his colleagues did not take the time to "lay the groundwork" for patients and their families to make thoughtful decisions about end-of-life care. Patients and families were also to blame, extending the principle of autonomy to "ridiculous extremes." "I can no longer separate what I do," he wrote, "from the totality of the patient's problems—the illness, the agony, the torture of a slow, but almost always, inevitable death, with the final months, weeks, days spent in the cold, artificial confines of the hospital, one of the most unpleasant situations I can imagine for such a purpose." To participate in such cases, he added, was "inhuman and morally wrong" as well as "professionally bankrupt."

As a result, my father increasingly viewed requests for antibiotic advice in such patients as misguided and instead asked *whether* such infections should be treated. Infection, he knew, was often the "final straw in the deterioration of so many of the body's vital organs and functions." Failing organs "encourage the growth of bacteria." In such terminal cases, even though a particular drug was available to treat a particular bacterium, that did not necessarily mean it should be used or given. Once my dad began to question the use of antibiotics in such cases, he also expressed reservations about other, even more aggressive interventions that were being undertaken.

It was no coincidence that my father's concerns about inappropriate end-of-life care became so passionate and angry in the early 1990s. Although the field of bioethics was two decades old and some of medicine's major transgressions—such as human experimentation without the subjects' consent—had been addressed, it was not until the late 1980s that doctors were forced to cede control of death and dying within hospitals. The first battleground had been in New York State in 1984, when a man discovered that physicians had let his hospitalized grandfather die of congestive heart failure instead of attempting to resuscitate him. It turned out that despite all of the new emphasis on patient autonomy, doctors had managed to retain control of the final chapter of life. Once revealed, however, this approach was no longer acceptable. In 1988, the New York state legislature passed the country's first do-not-resuscitate law. Other states quickly followed. Although the laws differed, the basic premise was the same: the patient or, in the case of incapacity, the family got to choose whether or not CPR was to be performed. More important, the default option was to resuscitate, regardless of the patient's condition.

As someone who was studying bioethics and would soon be teaching it, I believed that DNR laws were logical correctives to the often suffocating paternalism that had deprived dying patients of power for years. But as early as 1990, a backlash to the new autonomy emerged when Lawrence J. Schneiderman, Nancy S. Jecker, and Albert Jonsen published a paper entitled "Medical Futility: Its Meaning and Ethical Implications" in the June 15 issue of the *Annals of Internal Medicine*. The authors argued that, despite the wishes of patients and families, physicians were not obligated to provide futile care—such as CPR—that would not meaningfully improve patients' medical conditions. It was the doctors' equivalent of a Take Back the Night march, although, interestingly, of the three authors, only Schneiderman was a physician. Jonsen was my theologian mentor during my Seattle fellowship, and Jecker was a philosopher also on the faculty of the Department of Medical History and Ethics at the University of Washington.

The Schneiderman piece caused a great deal of controversy, and the *Annals* took the unusual step of publishing a second article in which the original authors detailed their critics' objections and then responded to them. Here were three highly respected bioethicists advocating that the decision-making authority just taken away from physicians be restored to them—albeit in carefully chosen situations. For my part, although I had the utmost respect for the authors and thought the article was well argued, I worried that their notion of medical futility opened the door for physicians to once again insert their own value judgments into patient care. In other words, it was better to discuss the concept of futile care with patients and families than to overrule them. Ultimately, this sort of reasoning won the day and the impact of the nascent futility movement proved to be limited.

As the *Annals* was one of the dozen or so medical journals that my father read, he saw the Schneiderman article when it was published. He quickly became a supporter of the concept of medical futility, even contemplating whether he should devote his energies to becoming an activist in the field. The rampant misuse of technology was at times "criminal," he wrote. "I've participated in the horrible and cruel prolongation of a biologic life, of a person whose disease process is totally irreversible—irretrievably so—but sustainable by inappropriate technology." Not surprisingly, he was also highly disappointed in *Cruzan v. Missouri Department of Health*, a 1990 case in which the US Supreme Court upheld a Missouri law stating that, before the ventilator of a patient in a persistent vegetative state was discontinued, individual states could compel the family to produce "clear and convincing evidence" that the patient would not have wanted to be kept alive by medical technology.

My father's journals detail the exact sort of seemingly futile cases that he encountered. For example, one elderly demented patient had both a feeding tube and a tracheostomy, a hole in his windpipe that was connected to a ventilator and enabled him to breathe. Although the patient was "never going to get better or leave a hospital-type setting," according to my dad, "his family will not accept that reality and continues to pray for a miracle, which will not be forthcoming." In other instances, doctors were the culprits, as in the case of a woman who had an "absolutely rampaging lymphoma" and was "obviously terminal and slipping rapidly." Still, her hematologist was actively transfusing her with platelets, cell fragments that prevent bleeding. In reality, my father wrote, a brain hemorrhage due to her low platelet count "would have been the most merciful thing that could have happened to her and her family, to minimize her conscious suffering and their pain at her awareness of dying."

In another case, a Mount Sinai kidney specialist—who my father believed was a "master of his craft"—was planning to initiate hemodialysis on an eighty-five-year-old woman who had managed to live more than eight years with leukemia but had recently developed kidney failure and several other serious medical problems. Fortunately, however, "the good Lord intervened": the patient quickly died one weekend, thereby preventing the doctors from robbing her "of the dignity and independence she's maintained these many years." Was my dad correct? It is impossible to know, but he did not let the nephrologist off the hook, telling him that the patient's sudden death confirmed that dialysis would have been a mistake.

Another case that my father encountered was not at the Mount Sinai but in Philip Roth's 1991 book *Patrimony*, which he read during a visit to my home. Roth's elderly father, Herman, who had been diagnosed with an inoperable brain tumor, had carefully completed a living will stating that he did not want to go on a breathing machine in the case of impending death. Yet when the dying man arrived unconscious to the emergency room, the attending physician had urged the younger Roth to approve the use of a respirator. Not surprisingly, my father was livid. "The fact that our sophisticated world of instant communication cannot incorporate the final wishes of a dying man and his family," he wrote, "is an indictment of our approach to life and death." Happily, Herman Roth's wishes were ultimately honored.

There was one issue as to which my father was clearly right, twenty years ahead of most others: his objection to the use of percutaneous endoscopic gastrostomy (PEG) tubes to feed patients who had dementia, cancer, or other end-stage conditions and could no longer eat. His gripe was the same as with other technologies. Putting these stomach tubes into "elderly, totally incapacitated nursing home patients" prevented them from "dying in peace and dignity after a lifetime of earning the right to do so." Indeed, they wound up dying "more horrible deaths," with "flexion contractures of their limbs and festering and penetrating bedsores—skeletal and blank-eyed remnants of the vibrant alive people they once were."

If such language brought to mind victims of the Holocaust, it was not coincidental. In one journal entry, my father wrote: "I jokingly tell some of my associates that when the Nuremberg trials are reconvened, I will submit their names as 'war criminals'—but I am not entirely joking." He planned to ask the chairman of medicine to set up a committee to help patients, families, and doctors who were "too weak or insecure to reach these decisions on their own" decline PEGs when appropriate. By the early twenty-first century, my dad had been vindicated. There were definitive data indicating that such feeding tubes did not prolong the lives or alleviate the suffering of nursing-home patients. It was more appropriate and humane to simply let such individuals eat what they wanted and keep their mouths moist.

An excellent example of a case in which my father believed that the focus on a patient's infection entirely missed the bigger picture involved an elderly man who had been hospitalized for nearly six months after breaking his hip and who then experienced a cascade of complications, including infection after infection. "My role in all of this," my dad ruefully noted, "was to juggle his antibiotics, risk severe toxicities from the multitude of drugs employed and constantly re-adjust and re-dose according to the circumstances." My father was thrilled when the family finally acknowledged the reality of the situation and took the patient home to die, but he thought it should have happened much sooner. In contrast, he had nothing but the highest praise for Jacqueline Kennedy Onassis when it was announced in May 1994 that the former First Lady had declined treatment for pneumonia and returned home to die when doctors discovered that her aggressive lymphoma had spread to her liver. Her courageous decision, he wrote, had been a bookend to the "strength and remarkable behavior" that she had demonstrated at the time of John F. Kennedy's assassination.

When discussing these types of issues, my father and I were largely on the same wavelength. As a house officer during my rotations in the medical intensive care unit and elsewhere on the medical service, I, too, had been highly perturbed at what I believed was the inappropriate prolongation of life. But there was also a huge disconnect between the two of us. My remedy for correcting this problem was to apply the tenets of the new bioethics, working with both patients' families and physician colleagues. Leading bioethicists had developed sophisticated strategies, such as living wills and other advance directives, for addressing the goals of care in end-stage patients. In contrast, my father, trained in an era in which experienced, compassionate physicians took the bull by the horns, had little interest in negotiation and debate. He made no bones about what he thought of bioethics, even though I was working in the field. Ethicists, he wrote, are not "in a comparable position to those of us who actually watch the day-to-day, hour-by-hour pain and suffering of the hopelessly ill." Many, he added, hadn't the foggiest idea what *Primum non nocere* (First, do no harm) really meant.

Over the years, particular cases caused genuine disagreement between my father and me. We were always civil; the Lerners were not one of those families (the kind that exist in the movies, at least) who had screaming fights about right and wrong at the dinner table. But there was real conflict. One of our more memorable discussions concerned the legendary comedian George Burns, who shared a birthday with my son, Ben. Burns was turning one hundred on January 20, 1996, Ben's third birthday, and my parents were in town for Ben's party. At some point that day, my father posed the following theoretical question: If Burns suddenly had a massive heart attack and developed heart failure and kidney failure as a result, would I dialyze him? I said yes, assuming that Burns or his family wanted to give it a try. Patient autonomy and informed consent were central. My father did not entirely disagree but, predictably, was more concerned with the bigger picture. Was dialysis ever appropriate for centenarians? Wasn't it likely that Burns would be too sick to recover, thereby meaning that any use of dialysis, even if temporary, would merely prolong the dying process? Fortunately, from my dad's perspective, Burns died suddenly of cardiac arrest forty-nine days later, before the doctors could get to him.

We also quarreled over one of my patients, a woman with end-stage liver disease. Despite her severe illness, this woman genuinely hated to come to the doctor. When I made helpful suggestions about possible interventions to buy her some time, she was always polite but never really interested. She made it clear to me on several occasions that she understood her prognosis and had no interest in heroic interventions. As a result, I strongly encouraged her to fill out a health-care proxy form naming someone to make medical decisions for her if she became unable to do so. If she did not fill out the form, I explained, she might be subjected to unwanted interventions when she eventually deteriorated. My patient dutifully returned the form at her next visit, having selected her husband to be her proxy.

One morning, this patient arrived for a regularly scheduled appointment, and my secretary immediately sought me out to tell me that she did not look well. It was a correct assessment. The patient's blood pressure was extremely low. We rushed her to the emergency room, where it became clear that she had a severe blood infection. Given her liver disease, she was going to die, even if we placed her on a ventilator. I sought out her husband, who had come to the appointment with her, and asked him, as her health-care proxy, what we should do.

The husband, who I had not met before, responded angrily. He seemed not to understand the concept of a proxy and was appalled that I was suggesting that we not do everything to try to save his wife. Given this response, we intubated the patient and sent her to the MICU, where they gave her antibiotics as well as other medications, known as pressors, to increase her blood pressure. As predicted, nothing worked. She continued to deteriorate and died on a ventilator a few days later, in just the manner she had wished to avoid.

I made a point of telling my father about the case, both because it had been very disturbing to me and because of his growing interest in these types of situations. When I got to the part about the patient's husband insisting that his wife be intubated, he interrupted me.

"You told him that you couldn't do that, right?" he asked.

"No," I said.

"But she was *your* patient and had told you that she did not want heroics," he replied.

I went on to explain that while that was true, her husband was her proxy and was therefore ethically and legally empowered to make the decision, even though I believed it to be the wrong one.

My father knew all about health-care proxies. And he knew that the husband might have tried to sue the hospital if we had disregarded his wishes. So my dad clearly understood my reasoning. But I knew that he was disappointed in me. I had put logistical concerns in front of my patient's welfare. His provocative way of viewing the case was that, at least in this one instance, I had become one of those ethicists who did harm.

When my father was confronted with a similar situation, he acted very differently. This was the story that began this book, in which he actively obstructed the resuscitation of a patient who did not have a do-not-resuscitate order. Our most pointed exchange about bioethics and the changing world of medicine occurred when he told me what he had done.

Fortunately, my father documented the details of the patient's illness and his actions in a six-page typed document that he wrote in

October 1996—shortly after the event—and placed with his journals. The patient, who he described as elderly, had both severe arthritis and vascular disease. She had apparently not been out of bed for several years and had already been hospitalized at the Mount Sinai for several weeks. My father had been intimately involved in her care, treating several complicated infections. Since the woman was immobile and had a very poor appetite, she had developed massive tissue breakdown in the area of her lower back and buttocks. He vividly described her daily misery: "Every time this woman was moved or even touched, the raw denuded skin would be further abraded, bleed, and give her agonizing pain as the sheets or dressings pulled away." It was impossible, he added, to position her comfortably. The woman had already declined certain potentially lifesaving interventions, such as a PEG tube, indicating that she was well aware of the terminal nature of her condition. Her primary physician, however, had not used these decisions as an opportunity to clarify her larger treatment goals or the issue of resuscitation.

When my father's infectious diseases team first realized that the patient had died, he decided, "unilaterally and without any discussion," and in "total disregard of the concept of patient autonomy," not to call a code, which would have summoned the chest team to begin resuscitation efforts. But when he left the floor, other staff members had misgivings. A house officer called the patient's primary physician, who told him to call a code even though roughly ten minutes had elapsed. When my father heard the announcement on the overhead page system, he returned to the patient's room, "quickly dispersed this effort and chased everyone out of the room." It was during this period that he physically placed himself between the patient's body and those attempting to resuscitate her.

That my dad could essentially get away with aborting two resuscitations on a patient with no DNR order was a testament to the enormous respect and authority he had at his hospital. It was a throwback to the Osler and Loeb eras, when deference to the senior physician's judgment—even when it directly contradicted protocol—was the rule.

In justifying his actions as "correct and merciful," my father used familiar language. The patient's life was unbearable, her prognosis was terrible, and all efforts to reverse her deteriorating situation had been either fruitless or declined by her. "We were stymied and stumped and she was paying the price for our inability to reverse things," he wrote. In this rendition, the cardiac arrest was simply the natural progression of someone with her incurable illness. The patient was dying and then had died. Just because technology was available and the woman was in a hospital did not mean it should be used. My father was not given to proclamations, but here he made one. He had acted "in the name of common, ordinary humanity" and based on his "30+ years as a physician responsible for caring and relieving the pain of my patients who can't be cured." The nurses, he wrote, were in agreement with his actions, but some of his fellow physicians had objected on both ethical and legal grounds, fearing that such behavior could lead to malpractice lawsuits.

When my dad told me the story, it was a frightening and jarring moment. I was, in fact, firmly on the side of his physician colleagues. Even though I had enormous respect for his clinical expertise, his actions had been far too godlike for me. Certainly such behavior would never have been permitted at my hospital. Ever dutifully documenting major events in his journals, my father confirmed that during that conversation I had, indeed, been "aghast." I was sure enough of my position that when I first saw his notes on the case, which he entitled "A Criminal Act," I assumed he was referring to his own behavior as criminal—albeit justifiable, in his eyes. But in fact, what he was terming *criminal* was the notion of attempting to resuscitate such a patient, one "unfortunate enough to try and die in a modern American hospital who has failed to sign a piece of paper or verbally communicate what her life-ending story should be."

By the time of my father's dramatic intervention, I was back at Columbia, having become a faculty member there in 1993. I had finished my Clinical Scholars fellowship and completed my coursework toward my PhD in history. Between 1993 and 1996, I would write my dissertation, occasionally traveling back to Seattle for research and my dissertation defense. Columbia was the logical place for me to begin my career as an assistant professor interested in practicing internal medicine and studying and teaching the history of medicine. I was familiar with P&S and Presbyterian Hospital, and the Center for the Study of Society and Medicine, where I had already done research, seemed an appropriate home for my nonclinical activities.

There were two other propitious aspects to my new job. First, the Arnold P. Gold Foundation, an organization begun by a Columbia pediatric neurologist and his wife and devoted to promoting humanism in medicine, was looking to fund a young professor at P&S. I was fortunate enough to win the professorship and thus began a very fruitful interaction with Arnold and Sandra Gold and their friends Russell and Angelica Berrie. Among numerous other innovations, the Gold Foundation conceived of the idea of the now ubiquitous white-coat ceremony, during which incoming medical students are cloaked with white coats for the first time, take the oath of Hippocrates, and are introduced to humanistic medicine. Second, although David Rothman continued to teach some bioethics, there were numerous opportunities for me to expand the curriculum for both medical students and house officers.

One of the first programs I initiated was the ethics and professionalism lunches for third-year medical students doing their rotations in internal medicine. These sessions drew explicitly on cases and situations that they were encountering during their clinical rotations. I had experienced many of them myself. So we discussed the right of medical students to learn procedures on patients and whether students were obligated to tell these patients they were just learning. I asked them about being grilled by more senior physicians on rounds or in the operating room, a practice dubbed *pimping*, which some educators had criticized. I mentioned that, as a student, I enjoyed getting asked about famous surgeons but realized that perpetually putting students on the spot could approach harassment. I also encouraged the students to speak up when they witnessed unethical behavior, particularly when it involved patients—exactly what I had not done when I was in their shoes.

Many of the scenarios I raised explicitly contrasted the old paternalism model with the new emphasis on patient autonomy. For
example, adult children of cancer patients at times requested that
the doctors not tell their parents the actual diagnosis, trying to emulate the benevolent deception that was so common in the 1950s and
1960s. But, I explained, recent studies had overwhelmingly showed
that people want to know they have cancer, even if it is terminal. The
students and I discussed ways to broach the issue with patients before
their families attempted to intervene. Another good example involved
the issue of doing an HIV test on a reluctant patient if a medical student or other hospital employee had been stuck with a needle while
drawing blood from him or her. When I was a house officer, if that
happened and the patient refused testing, we quietly drew an extra
tube of blood and whisked it to the laboratory, unlabeled, to find out
if the person was HIV-positive. But as of in the 1990s, New York
State law—on the basis of autonomy—had declared the patient's refusal of such testing to be inviolate. As a result, needlestick victims
actually went on a complicated mixture of anti-HIV medications
prophylactically until they were sure they were safe. Understandably,
many students were outraged. This was, I admitted, patients' rights
at its most vigorous and problematic.

Two topics I always covered were DNR orders and medical futility. Although I always taught the current legal and ethical norms, I
liked to pepper my presentations with some of my own cases that
challenged standard assumptions. For example, we discussed slow
codes, halfhearted resuscitation efforts that had been very common
when I was a medical student and resident but had subsequently become much rarer due to the objections of bioethicists. In one case,
I had actually seen medications injected into the mattress instead of
the patient, so determined was the supervising physician to let the
extremely end-stage patient die in peace. It was not that this doctor
was opposed to patient autonomy, I told the students, but he believed that the patient's family members had no idea what it meant
when they told the medical staff to do everything for the patient.
It was here that I might tell the story of the twice-foiled resuscitation of the arthritis patient, saving until the end the detail that the

physician in question was my father. I would joke that all doctors are closet paternalists (or, in the case of women physicians, closet maternalists). My father, of course, was out of the closet.

In addition to running these lunches, I also helped organize a Gold Foundation lunch series for the Department of Medicine interns and, with the help of Columbia nephrologist Jay Meltzer and the local Vidda and Rudin Foundations, a medical-ethics fellowship for third-year residents. In all of these venues, issues that my father encountered regularly came up: What was the best way to break bad news to a patient? How should physicians deal with difficult patients? Was it ever appropriate to mislead patients in order to provide hope or get them to cooperate? Should doctors give medical advice to family and friends? Should pharmaceutical representatives, like those who had pitched their products to my dad, be allowed to take medical students and residents out to lunch, or did that compromise the objectivity of young physicians? And, finally, should medical errors be concealed or revealed?

My father had struggled with this last issue as a consultant called into cases in which earlier medical care had been questionable. He had entertained the idea of disclosing such information to patients and family members but, as far as I could tell, had largely kept quiet. Most bioethicists, steeped in the philosophy of patients' rights and the importance of "doing unto others as you would have others do to you," increasingly advocated truth-telling in such situations. Not only did patients deserve this information, but some studies suggested that such admissions actually *lowered* the chances of a lawsuit. And after the Institute of Medicine reported that up to one hundred thousand patients died each year as a result of medical mistakes, this topic could no longer be brushed under the rug.

Of course, it was much easier to promote widespread discussion of errors around a conference table than it was to carry out the actual disclosure in the clinic or the hospital. But I tried to do so whenever I could. In one instance, I had left on a Thursday night for a long weekend after seeing a patient in clinic who had a fever and abdominal pain. I ordered blood tests for her but did not check them because I had gotten her a follow-up appointment with a surgeon on Friday morning and I assumed the surgeon would look at the laboratory work. The surgeon saw the patient and gave her oral antibiotics to take at home, but she did not check the test results, which were extremely abnormal and mandated admission to the hospital. The next day, the patient experienced worsening abdominal pain and came to the emergency room, where doctors diagnosed a ruptured abscess. She had successful emergency surgery but an extremely rocky postoperative course, almost dying on one occasion.

At some point, I called the surgeon. I suggested that we had both made an error and needed to tell the patient. We agreed to speak with her separately. I told the patient exactly what had happened, that I had made a mistake in assuming her blood tests would be checked and that I was sorry. She was surprised when she learned the details but appreciated what I had said. I then asked her if she would be willing to tell her story to students studying the topic of medical errors. She said yes, and over the years, she joined me several times. I emphasized to the students that this type of disclosure was quite a new phenomenon. It was difficult and was a skill that needed to be learned from experts and more senior colleagues, but it was the right thing to do.

I also reminded both students and residents that, although I taught them about the doctor-patient relationship, I had learned a lot from other physicians who were especially adept and empathic when it came to patient care. In fact, some of these teachers had been more junior physicians. In one memorable instance, we were gathered around the bedside of a severely ill patient. The patient's wife, who was standing with us, happened to notice a pin on the white coat of the senior resident.

"My husband belongs to that same organization," she informed the resident.

Without missing a beat, the resident removed her pin and affixed it to the patient's hospital gown. The gesture was so spontaneous and so warm that the woman began to cry. I was proud of the resident, and I tucked the memory into my back pocket.

One topic that I particularly liked to discuss was physician prestige. Should being an excellent doctor, especially one who makes less money and works longer hours than peers in other fields, allow someone to feel a sense of entitlement? Each year I showed the entering class of medical students a clip from the Hollywood film *The Doctor*, in which William Hurt plays a talented, but arrogant, surgeon. In one scene, Hurt's character impatiently gestures for the hospital chaplain to leave a patient's bedside. "Do some doctors actually think of themselves as more important than God?" I would ask the students. I also told them about a senior Columbia surgeon who had thrown a tantrum and severely injured his foot when a security guard would not let him enter the hospital without his ID tag, which he had left at home. The doctor had been called in at night to perform emergency surgery, and there he was, stuck in the hospital lobby. Who had been out of line here? And what about me? I liked to assign an essay I had written for the *New York Times* in which I sheepishly admitted to having jumped the queue in front of other hospital employees in order to get a flu shot more quickly.

These were issues that students and residents thought about, especially since they were the beneficiaries of Sidney Zion's campaign to reduce work hours. Was it still possible to be a great doctor if you worked fewer than eighty hours a week and never more than twenty-four hours at one time? What should you do if your patients were unstable but you were told to leave the hospital and hand over care to someone who did not know them as well? Was it truly possible to bond with patients given such restrictions? Did it matter that new doctors in training—in contrast to my father and myself—would never witness the evolution of a patient's illness over the crucial first thirty-six hours? Did being a great doctor entail constant devotion to one's patients and one's craft, or was it better to have outside interests and spend substantial time with one's family?

Teaching such provocative topics was great fun. It was also pretty easy for me. I was well versed in the relevant scientific, historical, and lay literature on these subjects and had plenty of personal anecdotes to tell.

It was not until I immersed myself in my father's journals, however, that I really understood how dramatically the practice of medicine had evolved over only a few decades. As a historian, I knew that such change was inevitable and that much progress had occurred. I also remained comfortable criticizing many of the decisions made by my father's generation of physicians. But situating myself in the middle of my dad's cases exposed me to an intoxicating type of medical practice that surprised me in the force of its appeal and eventually led me to revisit some very basic assumptions.

CHAPTER SIX

Treating the Whole Patient

As someone who was involved in promoting humanism in medicine and the doctor-patient relationship, I was well aware of several mantras: medicine had become too reliant on technology; doctors saw patients not as people but as specific diseases; physicians in training had become the equivalent of shift workers. Truth be told, I had heard the famous 1925 admonition by Harvard Medical School professor Francis Weld Peabody—"For the secret of the care of the patient is in caring for the patient"—so many times that it sounded almost hackneyed.

It was thus especially helpful for me to immerse myself in my father's accounts of some of his most challenging cases. Here was someone who had trained in an era when devotion to clinical knowledge and patient care was intrinsic to both medical education and practice. And my father, due to his upbringing, personality, choice of specialty, and job flexibility, had become an especially fervid patient advocate. I found that reviewing his cases, without really knowing what specifically had made him such an outstanding physician, was a huge eye-opener for me—even though I was also a physician as well as a humanist.

The patients I encountered in my dad's consultation files from the 1960s and 1970s, some of whom I mentioned in the second chapter, gave me insights into a type of clinical practice I had never really experienced. Exploration of some of his later cases—from the early 1980s to the mid-1990s, around the time that he prevented the initiation of CPR—provided even more intense revelations. The cases varied in certain ways. For example, as time went on, my father had to pay more attention to changing ethical norms that placed patients and families in charge of clinical decision making. But the cases all shared one characteristic: my father's intense engagement in both his patients' illnesses and lives. The more I read, the more I felt that the difference between my dad's medicine and mine was almost epistemological. I cared for patients and treated their diseases but did not know them as he did. What was the value of his superior knowledge? And what, if anything, did it entitle him to do as a patient's physician?

That several of his patients in the 1980s and 1990s had AIDS was particularly fitting. My father had entered infectious diseases during its early, heroic phase, just a few years after his mentors had been forced to watch young, vibrant patients dying of untreatable infections. Now, with the advent of AIDS, the same thing was happening. As my father approached his late fifties, he encountered perhaps the most challenging patients of his career. They tested both his scientific acumen and his skills at interacting with patients and families. When I opened one of his journals, a photograph of one of his AIDS patients, a gift from the man's parents after their son died, fell out.

I certainly knew one case that I would find in my dad's journals, perhaps his most memorable patient. Laura (not her real name) was a married woman in her twenties with two children who developed an extremely complicated and ill-defined disorder of her bone marrow and immune system in the mid-1970s. My father had become involved because she originally came to the hospital with the diagnosis of infectious mononucleosis (which turned out to be incorrect). Eventually, there would be many actual infections for him to treat. But he stayed involved—and essentially became Laura's primary doctor—because he bonded with her as a friend. Although I understood very little about her medical condition, and I heard about her less after I went to college, her ups and downs were well known to my mother, my sister, and me. Certainly, my father was always in a better mood when she was doing well.

The actual details of Laura's illness are less important than my father's intense involvement in the case. He did literature searches in areas far afield from his own specialty, encountering new diseases that had not been identified when he was in medical school. He contacted pathologists and other physicians at the New England Medical Center, Memorial Sloan-Kettering Cancer Center, the Cleveland Clinic, and other hospitals, asking them to review Laura's slides and her case to try to make a firm diagnosis. But most of all, he spent almost five years orchestrating Laura's care, initiating experimental treatments, trying to alleviate her pain and suffering, and giving her full access to himself, day or night. "This young lady is a very special person," he explained to the author of a book on the spleen to whom he wrote for advice, "and I would like to leave no stone unturned or potential lead unexplored in order to resolve her problem."

Throughout the early years of Laura's illness, her main complaint was headaches. Expert after expert could find neither a cause for her symptoms nor a particularly effective treatment. When one neurologist suggested that her headaches might be psychological in origin, given the stress of her condition, my father was uncomfortable. "[Laura] has been an exemplary patient," he wrote, "who has never exaggerated or over-emphasized any of her very significant complaints, and I must therefore give her the benefit of the doubt in this search for the cause of her headaches."

The inability to alleviate her headaches through traditional means led him to initiate a series of experimental therapies. What was most notable about this effort was that the proposed solutions were based on deduction, a series of hypotheses constructed by my father and other doctors grounded in the existing literature and their years of clinical experience and then applied to Laura's specific case. For example, when Laura was found to have an increased blood volume and too much of a particular protein, she received plasmapheresis, a process in which her blood was removed, treated, and replaced. The headaches improved for a while.

Later, Laura began an immunosuppressive drug, Cytoxan, given to her in the hope that it would suppress her overactive immune system. In this instance, my father took the interesting step of crafting a consent form for Laura to sign. In the late 1970s, consent forms for medical procedures, which had previously been obtained only before operations and sounded more like indemnity forms designed to get hospitals off the hook for bad outcomes, were becoming more commonplace. As patients began playing more active roles in their care, it made sense to formally document their willingness to undergo specific treatments, particularly those that were unproven or risky. Using immunosuppression for Laura's ill-defined condition was both. My dad knew that pure paternalism—in which the kind, all-knowing doctor kept the patient blissfully ignorant—was no longer acceptable.

The consent form underscored how intensely engaged my father was in Laura's case. It was a two-page single-spaced document that explained what the doctors had concluded about her condition and the risks and benefits of trying immunosuppression. "There is no specific drug for turning off the overactivity of my lymphocytes and there is no consensus of opinion as to the best drug for this purpose," the form read. "Dr. Lerner has selected Cytoxan based on its benefits in a totally unrelated but probably immunologic disorder called Wegener's granulomatosis." Both Laura and her husband signed the form.

Owing to the complicated nature of Laura's illness, she saw numerous doctors. My father always sent them notes as to his whereabouts and how he could be reached to discuss her case. These included his office numbers, our home number, and our contact information when we were on vacation. He also arranged an elaborate coverage system for Laura when he was away, particularly when she was not doing well.

Unfortunately, roughly five years after her initial presentation, Laura developed leukemia. My father and his colleagues had always feared that her disease would eventually evolve into a malignancy, which Laura knew. At this point, standard chemotherapy was begun, but the prognosis was poor. Moreover, Laura was in a great deal of pain. My dad's notes indicate that he himself administered narcotic injections to alleviate her symptoms.

Eventually, Laura required admission to the hospital. Her leukemia had not responded to the treatment, and her bone marrow was full of abnormal cells. At this point, she developed infiltrates on her chest X-ray that looked like some type of pneumonia. Because the problem was an infection, what to do was my father's call. And he struggled mightily. Even if he could diagnose the infection and successfully treat it, all that was left was widespread cancer, which meant "severe, unrelenting, desperate bone pain, requiring morphine and stronger." While sitting in the doctors' lounge, he penned a note in one of his journals: "Pain or life? I really don't know at this moment."

My father also acknowledged some misgivings with his extreme involvement in Laura's case. "I'm too close, too involved," he wrote. "She's like a relative, really. We've lived through this illness of hers together."

Ultimately, my father held off on prescribing antibiotics. But it turned out not to matter. Shortly after he wrote his note, Laura rapidly deteriorated and died. Somewhat surprisingly, I did not find any subsequent journal entries summarizing his experiences with Laura other than one brief note indicating that he had attended her funeral.

In hindsight, thirty years later, what could I conclude from Laura's case? For one thing, it was highly atypical. The inability of top doctors from across the country to reach a diagnosis was exceptional. In addition, no matter how devoted a doctor my father was, he could not have given this much time and energy to all of his cases. Finally, Laura was obviously a particularly motivated patient and an impressive person.

But what struck me most was my father's total immersion in not only her disease but her quest to get well. That is, as long as Laura was game, he was willing to explore every single option and provide every last bit of support that he could. Moreover, he did so by blurring conventional understandings of medical specialties and medication options, crafting a unique plan of treatment culled from his vast clinical knowledge and that of his peers. It is impossible to know the exact impact of my father's ministrations on Laura's survival, but I would like to think she knew that she was receiving all the expertise and comfort that was humanly available to her.

As Laura was dying, my dad was involved in a similar case, that of an older woman with leukemia whom I will call Susan. As with Laura, the patient's primary illness was not infectious in nature, but my father had been called in for periodic consults. Once the leukemia worsened and the infections became more frequent, he became engrossed. The dynamic with Susan differed from what he had with Laura. While Laura had been a trouper, Susan was frustrated and angry with her disease, which she survived for more than nine years. And my father became the receptacle for her vitriol. "She screams and carries on when the going gets tough," he wrote, "knowing that I understand and will never reproach her, never abandon her, *whatever!*" He even encouraged her to use him in this manner, suspecting that once she was drained, she became more rational, placid, and cooperative regarding treatment decisions. My dad suspected that his medical expertise had prolonged her life but was even surer that he had helped her mental suffering by letting her know that he "was *always* available, even for the most trivial of problems or questions." Susan was well aware that such a doctor-patient relationship was highly atypical. At one point, she remarked to my father that it was more like a parent-child interaction, even though she was considerably older than he was. Ever the paternalist, he did not seem to mind.

In Susan's case, there was an additional tie between doctor and patient. Susan had been one of my sister Dana's high-school teachers. In the summer of 1984, near the final stages of Susan's illness, Dana and my mother visited Susan at her apartment. Subsequently, my father noted in a journal entry, Dana and Susan exchanged "touching" letters. This story proved that the apple does not fall far from the tree—my sister later became a psychotherapist—but it also reminded me of a gesture I had heard about that surely belonged to an earlier era: physicians who brought their families on rounds in the hospital to meet their favorite patients.

Today, these types of personal encounters happen very rarely. I recall being involved in a discussion once about whether it was appropriate for physicians to hang pictures of their families in their offices. Doing so, some thought, was not good for maintaining professional boundaries; patients might ask intrusive questions. Of course, with Susan, the fact that my sister was her former pupil made such a visit more logical. But even if this had not been the case, would it have been so bad? Susan had never married and had no children. For over nine years, she was in constant communication with my father, who probably would have discussed his family with her even if she had not known Dana. Introducing everybody might have made perfect sense. Susan, he wrote, "has crossed over—she is no longer just my patient." As with Laura, she had become not only a friend but a dear friend.

What was also apparent in cases like Susan's was just how much influence my father had at the end of such patients' lives. Just as he had debated whether or not to treat Laura's last infection, he anticipated a similar circumstance arising with Susan. "I truly find," he wrote, "that I am literally in the position of determining when (and often how) a patient will die."

My father was profoundly ambivalent about such a task. Although he had an excellent sense of what a particular antibiotic could achieve in a particular situation and was willing to make hard choices, it was burdensome to be the one so often making such life-and-death decisions. So when Susan died, during my parents' annual vacation to France, my dad acknowledged that it may have been for the best that he was not at home. He did, however, regret missing the funeral.

As would be expected, my father's most intense patient interactions during these years usually involved chronically ill patients who had experienced recurrent infections over a prolonged period. But, as he did in his early years as a consultant, he continued to step in not only as a specialist but also as a caring doctor sensing a patient in need. One day in 1989, for example, he sat down and held the hand of a fifty-six-year-old man with cancer to give him "the reassuring words he desperately needs to carry on." My father explained that he "mustn't give up hope yet," as his upcoming chemotherapy was likely to help him. As someone who teaches the doctor-patient relationship, I wish my students could have been flies on the wall that day, watching a full professor and infectious diseases consultant taking time out of his busy day to offer a hand and an ear to a frightened cancer patient.

Not all of my father's patients in this era had terminal illnesses, although it almost seems like it from reading his journals. Occasionally, he included entries on patients who had recovered after infections. As usual, his scientific knowledge coupled with his insights into his patients helped him display keen clinical judgment. One such patient was a young woman with Crohn's disease, a type of chronic inflammation of the intestines. My dad had met her when an abscess in her pelvis spread to her brain, causing the formation of six smaller abscesses there, as well as the development of meningitis. She was extremely ill. The treatment for abscesses is to drain them and then give antibiotics, and that is what was done for the patient's pelvic infection. But my father decided not to have the neurosurgeons drain the brain abscesses, instead treating them with medication alone.

The basis of his decision? Fortunately, my father kept in one of his folders the scientific literature he had consulted during this case. Most heavily highlighted was an article entitled "Successful Treatment of Multiple Brain Abscesses with Antibiotics Alone," published in the *Reviews of Infectious Diseases* in 1985. There were only seven cases described in the article and they had been reviewed retrospectively, making it the exact sort of study that was falling out of favor in an era of sophisticated randomized controlled trials. But as an author of detailed clinical review articles, my father relied on them. The 1985 piece was apparently enough to convince him that it was reasonable to send the neurosurgeon away. My dad's treatment proved correct. The patient received several weeks of antimicrobials in the hospital and then was discharged.

But even this relatively brief encounter caused a lasting bond between doctor and patient. Several months later, ominously, the fluid in the pelvis returned. The fear was that it was another abscess that might again spread elsewhere in the body. Another drainage procedure was planned using an ultrasound machine for guidance.

My father had made time to go to the ultrasound suite, although he was not involved in doing the drainage. He wanted to watch the procedure for medical purposes and to provide emotional support to his patient. What happened next, my father wrote, was a "minor miracle": the fluid collection seen earlier in the week had disappeared. "Ecstatic," he kissed the patient on her forehead, hugged her mother, and told her story throughout the hospital all day.

As my dad dealt with these challenging cases, he also began to confront a new disease that was baffling and devastating. The AIDS epidemic that I first encountered in New York in the mid-1980s arrived in Cleveland at the end of the decade. As was true for his infectious diseases counterparts across the country, my father found that this awful disease gave him the opportunity to be a master physician, making difficult diagnoses as well as nuanced and elegant decisions about which antimicrobial agents to use. But even though these efforts resulted in some temporary successes, he knew that the vast majority of AIDS patients were fated to go downhill—and often very quickly. "I find these cases most painful," he noted, "because it's now an inevitable course we observe with only some little hope for slowing things down." An untreatable infectious disease that killed previously healthy young people within weeks or months, my father wrote in 1991, was a "frightening throwback" to a time "when there was nothing to do but watch death come in the door and take over the remaining months." How helpless and frustrated those doctors must have felt, he added, having only symptomatic treatments at their disposal. Not surprisingly, AIDS became a test case for my dad's support of medical futility. "Personally," he wrote, "I feel that heroic treatment of end-stage AIDS is morally wrong."

This did not mean, however, that my father was not up for the challenge of preserving some quality time for his AIDS patients. Using his tried-and-true techniques for engaging patients, such as spending extra time with them and explaining their illnesses, he got them to come to follow-up appointments and cooperate with in-hospital interventions, many of which were quite invasive. This success extended to several patients who had initially demonstrated "hostile, denial-based behavior."

Reflecting on these cases, my father explained his strategy:

I held nothing back. I made no promises but I convinced these patients that the situation was far from hopeless these days, that I was
very concerned that they understood the consequences of not ad-
hering to treatment, and that I was willing to do everything I could,
including working them into research protocols at the University,
to treat them and follow them on a long-term basis, so long as they
understood it was a two-way responsibility.

Building on the efforts of earlier breast-cancer activists, people
with AIDS took patient autonomy to new heights in the 1980s, demanding entrance into clinical trials and often knowing the scientific
literature better than their physicians. In some sense, they were the
embodiment of the new bioethics. My father's interactions with his
AIDS patients did not necessarily preclude such an approach, as seen
by his willingness to foster experimental treatments. But as I read
my dad's words, I felt they embodied the exact type of paternalism
that was in the process of being overthrown. "Trapped in a desperate
situation," he wrote, AIDS patients needed a "firm but concerned
individual to take charge of their health-related problems."

As was the case with Laura and Susan, my father developed very
intense relationships with several of his AIDS patients who he followed closely for months and, in a couple of fortunate cases, years.
As they finally deteriorated and neared death, he faced similar issues
about when to pull back—and about who should decide.

One of my father's first patients with AIDS was Michael, who
he later described as a "slim, handsome young man, with a grace-
ful walk and beautiful skin." Unfortunately, Michael was a textbook
example of the devastating and widespread infections that AIDS
patients could get. These included the fungal infection histoplas-
mosis, which caused him severe pneumonias and a collapsed lung;
the parasitic infection toxoplasmosis, which caused tumors in his
brain; and the viral infection cytomegalovirus, which caused an infection of the retina that eventually took Michael's vision. Admitting
that infectious diseases doctors "did not yet know how to treat the

opportunistic infections of AIDS too well," my father nevertheless successfully juggled antibiotics in a way that kept Michael out of the hospital for prolonged periods.

As would be expected, my dad once again went the extra distance, visiting Michael at his home every Sunday morning. It was not an easy thing to do. One Sunday, his patient was doing well enough that my father took a day off. "I am thankful I didn't have to go today," he wrote, "as it drains me to do so." He benefited greatly from the help of his Mount Sinai colleagues, especially the nurses, who he later praised in his journals. The nursing staff, he wrote, "was remarkably compassionate and not frightened by his diagnosis."

One month later, Michael was worse. Writing early one morning, my father announced that he "could no longer, in good conscience, recommend continuing treatment." Poor Michael was paralyzed, blind, and demented. What was in store for him was a breathing tube in his windpipe, probable kidney failure, and a very toxic drug, amphotericin B—nicknamed "amphoterrible"—and then he would die anyway. "As physicians we are pledged to treat disease," my father wrote, "but when we have to admit that we can't win the struggle, why must we go through the motions nonetheless?" He planned, that very afternoon, to convince Michael's supportive and loving parents "to withdraw all of our treatments and let him go."

But Michael was young with a strong heart. He held on for another week or so, long enough for my parents to leave for their annual sojourn to France. The end went as smoothly as it could have; my father had left explicit instructions for the covering physicians. As in the case of Susan, he regretted not being in town for Michael's death and funeral, but it was also a blessing for him to be away. Still, sitting on my uncle's terrace, he rebuked himself for not having pressured Michael's parents to cut back earlier, worrying that he had taken the easy way out.

In 1989, my dad saw another AIDS patient in consultation. Hospitalized in an intensive care unit on Cleveland's west side, the man was running a very high fever for which no specific cause had been found. He already had an excellent infectious diseases consultant, but the family wanted a second opinion and reassurance that nothing was being overlooked in the case. Unable to free up time during the week, my father did the consultation on a Saturday morning. He allotted three hours to do "a proper job." Believing that an underlying cancer was a "good bet," he made a few recommendations to the doctors. Later that afternoon, he reflected on the experience. Whether the patient did or did not have an infection seemed almost irrelevant: "Here is a handsome young man," he wrote, "twenty-four years of age, with tubes coming out of his chest, on a respirator, wasted and pale, anxious and frightened, who is going to be dead soon and there is no way I or anyone else is going to prevent that inevitability." My father did not mention meeting the family, but I suspect that if he did, he spent as much time discussing their heartache as he did talking about the medical details he had been asked to elucidate.

Meanwhile, my father was taking care of another AIDS patient at the Mount Sinai. In contrast to the situation a couple of years earlier, infectious diseases specialists had learned how to better treat the opportunistic infections associated with AIDS. So in the case of a man I will call Larry, my dad was able to keep him alive for close to three years, even deluding himself at one point that his patient might "beat the odds." Like many such patients, Larry eventually developed Kaposi's sarcoma, a rare and incurable cancer found predominantly in the skin and other organs of immunocompromised patients.

At first, my father did not mention the Kaposi's to Larry. It was his usual paternalism. As there was nothing to do right away, why upset his patient, who was maintaining a stable weight and even going to the gym? All along, without denying the reality of AIDS, my father had been "trying to paint as rosy a picture as I could." But eventually he ordered skin and lymph node biopsies, which confirmed the diagnosis of Kaposi's. When the results came back, he told Larry that his remaining time was limited. This led to the next decision point: Should my dad and his colleagues initiate chemotherapy, which was both highly toxic and unproven in the case of Kaposi's, to give Larry some continued hope?

In this instance, Larry—in conjunction with his parents, whom my father got to know very well—made the call: they wanted to do everything. Chemotherapy was begun. Two subsequent pneumonias were successfully treated. But by this point, it was clear that the Kaposi's had spread to Larry's lungs. He was dying.

It was time, my father knew, for a frank talk. Although he would have been perfectly content to merely quietly withhold resuscitation and artificial ventilation from Larry when the time came, my father knew he was dealing with a patient and family who embodied the new spirit of autonomy. So he had the exact sort of end-of-life discussion that I taught medical students and residents at Columbia to have. If it was overwhelmingly likely that resuscitation would not work and Larry would die on a ventilator in an intensive care unit, would he still choose that option? Larry not only said yes but, according to my dad, was somewhat angry at the question and concerned that the doctors were giving up on him.

In an interesting twist of fate, my father was at the Mount Sinai one Saturday night when Larry, dramatically short of breath from yet another bout of pneumonia, arrived at the hospital. Attending physicians were covering the patients so the house staff could attend an annual party in their honor. The vast majority of those working were young, having recently completed residency themselves. But in arranging coverage for the event, the residents knew if they asked my fifty-eight-year-old father, he would probably say yes. And he did.

So when it was time to choose whether to intubate Larry or let him die, it was my father, respecting his patient's wishes, who put him on a ventilator and sent him to the intensive care unit. "It was my worst nightmare, and it came true," he later wrote. "It was something I didn't want to do and something that could easily be argued was wrong to do (morally and ethically), but, nonetheless, I did it."

Larry lived for six days. Unable to talk while on the ventilator, he eventually wrote my father a note saying he did not want CPR. So when Larry continued to deteriorate, he was allowed to die, comfortable and surrounded by his loved ones.

Despite his great opposition to futile treatment and the fact that he had known Larry would not make it, my father did not regret what had happened. Larry had staged a "magnificent last stand": he "left no stone unturned and was determined to battle this illness with everything he could muster and his determination never faltered." My father was also pleased that he was able to spend some quality time with Larry during his last days, less as his physician than as a "concerned friend." Larry died in the manner that he had wished.

As I tried to process in my mind all of my dad's efforts to not prolong—and occasionally to speed—the deaths of his end-stage patients and relatives, it was reassuring to see him pause and at least contemplate other options. Even the best physicians need to adapt to changing times. Larry's parents were pleased with what had transpired. At the funeral, they asked my father to sit with them. "I was very touched," he wrote. After the burial, my father and his secretary, Shirley, returned to the church for lunch, where they heard many stories about Larry and "got to know him much better." Thus began "the age-old process of healing." My father also noted that Larry's parents occasionally "dropped by to say hello" to him for a couple of years after their son's death, an important step in their mourning process with which he was pleased to assist.

My father's most intense experience with an AIDS patient was a man I'll call Jonathan, a patient who arrived at the Mount Sinai in late 1991 in terrible shape, having already had life-threatening pneumocystis pneumonia that had decimated both of his lungs. He had essentially no CD4 cells to fight infections. My father placed Jonathan on an extremely complicated fifteen- to twenty-pill regimen, including azidothymidine (AZT), then the only effective treatment for HIV infection, and an experimental drug to prevent a lung infection common in AIDS patients. Nevertheless, about a year into Jonathan's treatment, he had developed an "unrelenting fever" that was possibly being caused by an undiagnosed cancer. "How hard should I push?" my dad asked himself.

With the encouragement of his patient and his patient's parents, my father pushed hard. He and his Mount Sinai colleagues, including my uncle Allan, kept Jonathan alive and mostly out of the hospital for almost two and a half years. It was, my father wrote on the day of Jonathan's death, "an odyssey . . . an incredible and epic struggle to plug the dike each time a leak appeared." Among the conditions my dad treated were pancreatitis, peripheral neuropathy (arm and leg numbness), severe leukopenia (low white blood cell count), and anemia. As Michael had, Jonathan developed cyto-megalovirus retinitis, cerebral toxoplasmosis, and several other in-fections. Although my father modestly wrote that he was mostly providing "friendship and cheerful support," he managed these con-ditions with his usual legerdemain, using approved and unapproved medications and improvising when earlier strategies failed. Sensing that Jonathan was holding too many of his emotions inside, my fa-ther urged him, albeit without success, to see a psychologist. But in 1994, an enlarging spleen proved to be an insurmountable problem. My father had concluded that the undiagnosed cancer causing the elevated temperatures was likely a lymphoma that was growing in Jonathan's spleen and elsewhere. Moreover, the growing spleen was causing substantial pain, something that the patient had somehow been spared until that point. There was also new fluid in Jonathan's abdomen, a condition known as ascites, suggesting that the cancer might have also spread there.

It was another "How hard should I push?" moment. This time, my father held back. Chemotherapy, he believed, "would be too difficult for him to tolerate," and "lymphomas, in this setting, are notoriously resistant anyway." When he admitted Jonathan to the hospital for the last time, the main medication the patient received was intrave-nous morphine for his pain. Jonathan died several days later.

How did my dad reach this decision? One thing he did not do was explicitly ask his patient's opinion. There was a different dy-namic here than there had been with Larry. All along, my father and Jonathan had discussed his reaching a point when there were no more "corners to turn." At such a time, my dad believed, he and Jonathan had a "tacit understanding" that they would "proceed ac-cordingly." My father had mentioned the possibility of a lymphoma in the past, and the fact that Jonathan remained passive and asked no questions further convinced him to take charge. If one strictly ap-plied the teachings of bioethics and patient autonomy, as I did in the classroom and on the wards, Jonathan should have been formally apprised of the findings and asked about his choices. It would not have been particularly appropriate to ask Jonathan's parents what they wanted because he still had decision-making capacity. But my father did inform them of what he had decided, and they "agreed."

Phil Lerner was well aware that he was again in tricky territory. "I admit that this is medical paternalism at its very extreme," he wrote. But prolonging Jonathan's life, with a painful, cancerous spleen that could not be treated, made no sense. "I was determined not to let him suffer physical pain on top of the mental anguish he was experiencing," my father later wrote. In addition, Jonathan's parents "were spared a more prolonged period of watching their son die." My dad also penned the following: "I was able to use my skills as a physician to ease his passage, not my skills as a specialist to prolong his suffering." In another note, he went so far as to call what he had done "close to euthanasia," although most bioethicists would not have used that word to describe what occurred. Jonathan had died not from the morphine, which was appropriately used to control his pain, but from his underlying disease.

What made my father believe he had the authority to make these decisions? Once again, it was his immersion in the medical and emotional care of a patient over a prolonged period. During the two-plus years he cared for Jonathan, my dad often called his patient from meetings, and once, while flying to New Orleans, he even arranged for a special X-ray test to be done. There was always a contingency plan for Jonathan and his family if my father was out of town and could not easily be reached. "We became 'friends' in a sense," my father reflected.

Near the end, when Jonathan was on a respirator in the intensive care unit and beginning to fade, his doctor took his hand. "He squeezed my hand in return, as he smiled at me," my father wrote, "thanking me, I think, for being so concerned about him."

As would be expected, my father attended Jonathan's funeral, where his role in the case was praised by Jonathan's father. Later that day, he paid his condolences at the family's home, where he was able to speak to several of Jonathan's relatives. "I was particularly touched by his sister," my father wrote, "who embraced me with such a genuine show of affection for my role in her brother's illness that I felt she considered me a part of their family when it came to the mourning process I too needed to resolve." My dad was also especially pleased when he received a note from Jonathan's parents thanking him for the "gentle way" he helped their son die.

Reading my father's account of Jonathan's saga was a moving experience for me. Jonathan had died as a young man—he was only five years older than I—and of a terribly frightening and devastating disease. My father had given his patient terrific medical care and emotional support. Still, I was not prepared for what happened as I went through my father's journal entries: a photo of Jonathan, sent by his parents, dropped out. And there he was, in the flesh: a smiling, carefree man. On the back was a Post-it with a brief, typed note:

> phil:
> this was jonathan before he was stricken with aids.
> and, it's the way we will always remember him.

Of course, on second thought, I realized it made perfect sense. Why wouldn't Jonathan's parents want to send my father such a picture? And why wouldn't my father want to have it?

Reading about Jonathan's 1994 death made me reflect on the episode that occurred two years after, when my dad prevented CPR on the woman with arthritis. Could it be argued that in both instances, as well as with my father's other AIDS cases, there was a medical reality that actually enabled him to know the "right" decisions? By this I do not mean that there was only one possible course of action and that only my father knew it. But had medicine, in an era of patients' rights and splintered care, somehow become too democratized? And as a result, were patients routinely undergoing inappropriate interventions and experiencing needless suffering?

My father would have unswervingly answered yes to these questions. The theme of knowing came through constantly in his journals. Describing his reaction upon learning that Jonathan had developed an enlarged spleen and ascites, my father later wrote, "I knew that we now had to think only of keeping him comfortable." "I know what I did was right," he remarked after Jonathan died, "because all of my colleagues who helped me care for him—and there were many—were equally relieved that his suffering was over and the end came swiftly and peacefully." When discussing the demented patient who had feeding and breathing tubes and whose family was waiting for a miracle, my dad made his case most forcibly. "I know in my heart," he unabashedly declared, "when certain patients are ready to go."

Such language could not have been more reminiscent of some of the quotes from the breast surgeons and other postwar doctors I had researched. I had termed them *arrogant*, and my father sounded much the same. Yet maybe, as my father might have suggested, his obligation in both of these cases was exactly the same: to use his medical knowledge and his knowledge of the patient to do the right thing. Perhaps, to rewrite Peabody's old saw mentioned at the beginning of this chapter, the secret of the care of the patient was in learning as much as you could about the patient and his or her disease and dutifully using that knowledge to make the best choices for that person. The sociologist Charles Bosk has called this type of interaction the idealized fiduciary relationship between a powerful and devoted doctor and his or her patient.

In the prologue to this book, I mentioned a statement made by Columbia gastroenterologist Robert Whitlock in which he called Robert Loeb "the best damned ethicist I ever met." When I first heard this, I rolled my eyes. After all, Loeb, with his bullying of medical students and his imperious demeanor, embodied the exact sort of misguided physician authority that the bioethics movement had challenged.

But after reading my father's journals, I understood what Whitlock had meant. And I also knew why Saul Farber, the longtime head of medicine at New York University, rarely bothered to convene the hospital ethics committee that he chaired in the 1980s. If you practically lived in the hospital, knew the medical literature up and down, and placed the patient on a pedestal, how could you not make the most ethical decisions? Who needed ethical principles and patient-empowerment tools when the right answers were sitting there right in front of the compassionate doctor's nose? As my father wrote, becoming so immersed in his patients' cases and constantly interacting with their families made him "a much more aware and caring physician." Whether or not I could conceive of practicing medicine in this manner, it certainly was a compelling, and even heady, argument.

In addition to reflecting on my father's behavior from the perspective of a physician, I also did so as a historian. Placing his actions in historical context had been relatively easy. He had trained as a doctor at a time when paternalism by all-knowing, benevolent physicians was the norm. But what about my history? Whereas I thoroughly understood why historians and bioethicists had called into question the excesses and mistakes of my father and his peers, I had not fully historicized my own experiences. My education and training occurred during the ascendancy of patient autonomy, and many of my mentors had played major roles in promoting this concept. My beliefs, like my dad's, had been shaped by my history. From this perspective, it made perfect sense that I was now scrutinizing them.

My father's efforts to challenge the changing ethical norms surrounding death and dying did not stop with his arthritis patient. As of the mid-1990s, he was the de facto physician for three elderly relatives: his mother, his mother-in-law, and his aunt. Knowledge of one's patients' lives conveyed authority to a doctor, and my father knew these women as well as anyone he had ever treated. So when they grew increasingly ill, he took charge in a way that was, once again, simultaneously disturbing and humane.

CHAPTER SEVEN

Family Practitioner

It was not inevitable that my father would play such a major role in the care of his family members—becoming not only cousin Phillip but also Dr. Phillip. His gradual decision to do so was a function of the worrisome trends he saw in medicine: increasing bureaucratization; distancing of doctor and patient; and overreliance on technology, especially at the end of life. My dad had played auxiliary roles in the care of my grandfather Mannie and my mother in the 1970s, but both of these bouts of illness had been self-limited. However, when my aging relatives began to develop degenerative diseases and terminal cancers, my father's inclination to become involved grew— as with his uncle Mickey, who was dying as I began medical school.

Revisiting the stories of my father's legendary patients, both those with AIDS or other diseases, had been tricky enough. But the stories of his involvement—or over-involvement—in the care of relatives I had known for my whole life made things even more complicated. With all of the admonitions against physicians caring for their family members, was he being a good doctor? I needed to explore this question as a physician, a historian-ethicist, and, finally, a son.

Mickey, a lawyer in Cleveland, was actually only nine years older than my father, almost more of an older brother to him than an uncle. He was just fifty-nine years old when he became ill in the spring of 1982. The diagnosis was grim: pancreatic cancer that had already spread to the liver. My father had gone looking for the results of the diagnostic ultrasound, and, I learned from his journals, when he found them, he reacted to the grim news by kicking a chair in dismay. I also learned that he had been the one to tell Mickey both his diagnosis and that he was unlikely to live more than one year. My reflexive reaction to this revelation was negative—Mickey's doctor should have told him—but I knew this was only the beginning of my father's increasingly active role in caring for sick family members.

Mickey's decline was rapid. Within a few months, he was already in the terminal stages of the disease, in substantial pain and barely eating. When Mickey was admitted to the Mount Sinai Hospital in July 1982, my father visited him daily. As there were no issues of infection, he was not officially a part of the team, but he believed he could help make sure that Mickey was receiving adequate palliative care. But mostly, he came as a nephew.

Even though my father was accustomed to death and dying, it was what he called "a particularly difficult death." Most difficult was "the slow and painful (physically and psychically) deterioration of someone I truly loved." The fact that my father, such a capable doctor, was largely helpless in the face of the cancer only made things worse. "There were days when I was so depressed, I had to force myself to go to the hospital," he later wrote. "Nothing has ever drained me so thoroughly." Indeed, one day toward the very end, when Mickey was heavily sedated, my dad did not go visit. He felt less depressed but "terribly guilty."

Mickey died at four o'clock on a Friday afternoon, when my father was still at the hospital and other family members could quickly be assembled. His uncle had been "considerate, cooperative and uncomplaining to the very end," he remarked.

For my father, the death had not come soon enough. Mickey had suffered far too much. Ironically, shortly before Mickey died, we had decided to put down our beloved family dog Lily, who had experienced months of neurological degeneration leaving her nearly unable to walk. I had not yet left for medical school, and my father and I drove together to the veterinarian. I was far too upset to participate in the process so my dad, once again the family's doctor, took over, holding Lily in his arms as she received the fatal injection. I wonder why, my father wrote, "we could relieve the suffering of our animals with the snap of our fingers, but could not offer similar surcease, in some fashion, for our human loved ones." As my father became more and more engrossed in the topic of medical futility and more heavily involved in the deaths of my grandmothers, he actively sought to blur this line.

During the 1980s and 1990s, as my parents' relatives and friends aged, I often received reports on their medical conditions. This may be normal, to some degree, although my sister and I always found it rather morbid. But when it came to my father, medical updates were his lingua franca. Not surprisingly, the pages of his journals were filled with the illnesses and recoveries of people I knew very well, those I did not remember, and those I had never met. Even though the diseases they developed were mostly random, it was almost as if their illnesses provided a type of road map for their lives and, by extension, my family's. "It is difficult to know where to start," opened one 1987 journal entry addressed to my sister and me, "but I'd best recount the illnesses first." Reflecting on an elderly cousin in a nursing home with dementia, he recalled a photograph of a family gathering from the 1930s in which she looked "absolutely stunning." Her current condition was "in stark contrast to the memories and pictures of the past." About the death of a cousin's wife in 1985, he wrote that it "marks the beginning of a new transition, as I and my cousins enter the last stages of our lives." "The fragility of our life on this earth," he wrote after the unexpected death of a friend, "is periodically pointed out to us in these little events that remind us of our mortality." In 1992, he even composed a note detailing all of the cancers on his side of the family that had been diagnosed and treated at the Mount Sinai.

This tendency to obsess about the illnesses of others only accelerated when it came to discussions of my father's peers. The diseases that doctors developed seemed to hold some special symbolic value for my dad and other physicians of his generation. At my father's medical school reunions, it was routine for attendees to recount their medical ailments—in great detail—to their fellow classmates. One former classmate's tracheotomy, he wrote after a reunion, "tells a tragic tale unfolding." When I interviewed doctors for my books and asked them about their mentors, they often shook their heads sadly and told me what diseases had caused their deaths. It was almost as if these physicians, who had trained and practiced during medicine's golden age, when anything seemed possible, had seen themselves and their colleagues as somehow invulnerable. But they also appreciated that disease, as shown most vividly in the case of AIDS or cancer, remained a formidable adversary that deserved respect. When the doctor being discussed had died from the exact condition that he or she had researched and treated, which seemed to happen more often than expected, it was especially moving.

One journal entry, for example, described the unfortunate diagnosis of brain cancer in Harold Neu, the infectious diseases specialist who had been one of my professors at Columbia and who lived one block away from me in suburban Westchester County. "Harold," my father wrote, "is dying of an inoperable brain tumor but carrying on to the bitter end heroically." Remarkably, Neu actually lived for several years with his cancer, enabling my father to visit him at his home when he came to New York to see my sister and me. "Had a shock when I read of the tragic passing of Bernard Fields," read another journal entry, "the brilliant Harvard virologist at the age of 58 from pancreatic ca."

When a physician died while tending to patients, it was all the more tragic and meaningful. A journal entry dated November 26, 1993, told of the sudden death of one of my father's Mount Sinai internist colleagues during rounds at the hospital. This doctor had frequently come to the Mount Sinai at night and on weekends when his patients needed admission, even when he was not on call. It was not surprising that my father had so much admiration for this man, who, he wrote, represented "a dying breed, the indefatigable solo practitioner who knows all about his patients and follows them himself closely and confidently until their problems are resolved."

Depending on who the relatives or friends were, where they lived and what diseases they had, my father got involved in their care to different degrees. People loved to run cases by him, both because they trusted his medical judgment and because he knew almost the entire Cleveland medical community. On one occasion, when he went to see his mother, Pearl, who had fainted in her apartment, there were three people present who asked his medical advice on other issues. He was surely happy to provide it. It is not clear if there was a specific moment when my father decided to insert himself more directly into the care of certain relatives, but the reasons he did so seem clear. In an era of increasingly impersonal medical care, directed by doctors who were overextended and hassled by insurance companies and who practiced "cookbook" medicine, he thought he could help ensure that his loved ones received the individualized, hands-on attention that he had been taught to provide. Meanwhile, the notion that his dying relatives and friends might become the victims of futile treatment was entirely unacceptable. "My talents prolong the lives and sufferings of strangers," he wrote in 1991. "I would never do things like this to a loved one!" Finally, there were the themes that ran throughout his journals: his relatives had shown the courage to move to the United States, had nurtured my father, and had enabled him to achieve his dream of becoming a physician. How could he—their cousin, their nephew, their son— not pay them back?

It was this mind-set that led him to get highly involved with the care of one of his first cousins, Donald, who developed prostate cancer in the early 1990s. Donald, the son of one of my Grandma Pearl's sisters, was the first of his cousins living in Cleveland to become seriously ill. Donald was also our family accountant and, as my father often remarked in his journals, one of his favorite people. The turning point in Donald's case came in 1992, when he developed painful metastatic disease to his spine.

The timing was particularly poignant. In June 1992, when Donald made a casual remark to my dad about the gradual loss of Jewish traditions in the family, it had "triggered an idea": What if my father wrote a brief history of the Singers—Pearl's very large family— in time for a family reunion, planned for September of that year? Thus was born "Cousins: The Next Generation," a thirty-four-page booklet that recounted the journey of Chaim and Dina Singer from

Poland to the United States and the fate of their plentiful offspring, which included almost fifty great-grandchildren (one of whom was me). The final product was a labor of love, and not just for my father. Throughout the summer of 1992, he spent every Sunday morning with his mother, Pearl, picking her brain about her childhood and her relatives, dead and alive. He also asked his cousins to provide information about their branches of the family tree.

The final document, replete with stories and pictures, was a big hit with my father's cousins. I'm not sure if my generation found it as compelling, despite my dad's hope that "the strong sense of family recalled by the cousins will filter down to their children and grandchildren, since much has been lost or diluted, at least, by the passage of time and the dispersal geographically of the close-knit family from a tiny village in Poland." My father loved the reunion, which, he wrote, "recalled the family club picnics of my youth and an era of simpler times." I might have helped promote family unity by attending the reunion, but Cathy and I were living across the country in Seattle during my fellowship. In retrospect, having written this book, I wish I had made it my business to attend.

It was two weeks after the reunion that Donald called my father to tell him about the progression of his disease and to discuss an oncologist that he was planning to see. By December, Donald was traveling to Detroit to try a novel combination of chemotherapy drugs. My father was becoming increasingly involved in the case, helping Donald to get a series of studies he required before starting the chemotherapy. "He's only got a 30–50% chance of responding," he recorded in his journals.

Three months later, my dad was even more involved. "I suddenly find myself taking care of my cousin Donald," he wrote. He described how this had occurred. Donald's primary oncologist was in Detroit, and even though he also had one in Cleveland, Donald had let my father and his physician-brother, Allan, know that he was happy to rely on them for ongoing medical advice. This new responsibility was one reason that my parents canceled their annual trip to France. My father approached the task with trepidation. Although he was "glad to be able to help" because it gave Donald "a little more control" and allowed him to "avoid unnecessary treatments" and minimize visits to doctors, he feared that when Donald deteriorated, it might force my father "to make some hard decisions." Doing so as both a treating physician and a "cousin and good friend" was a potentially fraught conflict of interest.

The bioethicist in me, reading this passage, wishes my father had simply articulated these concerns to Donald and elicited his end-of-life preferences. Taking care of one's cousin was iffy enough. Indeed, this relationship probably made it even more crucial that the patient's autonomous wishes be identified and honored. But given my father's paternalistic leanings, this was unlikely to occur, at least while Donald remained semi-stable. Nor did Donald seem uncomfortable letting my father (and his brother) run the show.

Five months later, during the summer of 1993, Donald was much worse. His rapid deterioration, my father wrote, was "startling," even for someone like himself who had witnessed these types of cases many times before. By this point, Donald had made his wishes known: he wanted to die at home and not be readmitted to the hospital.

Even though the plan was to make Donald comfortable, my father was impatient. "I am most concerned that his suffering end as soon as possible," he wrote, "so we can remember him as he was, the Donald we all knew and loved so much, not the Donald who suffered so at the end." My dad planned to speak to Donald's wife and children "as soon as possible" to encourage them to ask Donald's Cleveland oncologist—who had once again become his primary physician—"to ease his way out of this terrible suffering."

As usual, with this sort of language, my father was pushing the envelope, suggesting a level of comfort with euthanasia that was not shared by most physicians or society. Ultimately, Donald availed himself of some of the evolving technologies for treating the pain of dying cancer patients, such as an indwelling epidural catheter used for administering strong analgesic medications. Happily, my father wrote after Donald's death, his final days had actually been quite peaceful, and his loving family had had ample time to say good-bye.

My parents had decided to euthanize our dog Lily shortly before Mickey's death, and, in an ironic twist, they had to put down Lily's successor, Sabine, just as Donald began to worsen. My father once again remarked on how dying animals experienced more humane deaths than humans did. Perhaps charting new territory in the world of bioethics—should doctors treat their own pets?—my dad had actually taken over Sabine's care after he grew impatient with the veterinarian's inclination to order additional tests for what was apparently a hormonal abnormality known as Cushing's disease. "I decided," he wrote, "after doing my own literature search, to initiate treatment myself." Although there was some initial improvement, Sabine later worsened.

It is hard not to think of Jack Kevorkian when reading my father's thoughts on death. Kevorkian was a pathologist who championed the rights of terminal patients to request assistance in dying. Between 1990 and 1998, it is estimated, he sped the deaths of 130 people. In order to ensure that patients themselves—as opposed to doctors—initiated the process of euthanasia, he developed machines that delivered lethal doses of gas or chemicals when the patient pressed a button.

Although he appeared to be an advocate of patients' rights and of death with dignity, two concepts promoted by bioethics, Kevorkian was loathed by most ethicists. First, by encouraging physicians to help patients kill themselves, Kevorkian was asking them to violate the Hippocratic oath, a section of which prohibited doctors from giving "deadly medicine." Second, investigations into Kevorkian's cases suggested that some of his patients had not been terminal and that others had not been appropriately referred for assessment of their psychiatric states or for pain management. Eventually, in 1999, a Michigan court convicted Kevorkian of second-degree homicide in conjunction with a death aired on TV's *60 Minutes*.

My father was no fan of Kevorkian either, criticizing his "misguided actions." But, he wrote, Kevorkian was "filling a major void in our society—the need to address the issue of death and dying." My dad favored legislation, which eventually passed in Oregon and a few other states, that legalized physician-assisted suicide, a carefully controlled process in which doctors could supply terminally ill patients with enough pills for them to end their lives at home.

It was more than just his cousin Donald that caused mortality to be on my father's mind. By the early 1990s, he was actively involved in the medical care of three octogenarians who were very dear to him and all of us: my grandmother Jessie (my mother's mother), my grandmother Pearl (my father's mother), and Aunt Gertie, my grandfather Meyer's older sister. Although he described them as "tough, stubborn, argumentative women" who "snipe and interrupt and expostulate," they were very much his "three angels."

In point of fact, all three women were in pretty good shape—"remarkably intact mentally, and even physically." Jessie was losing her vision and hearing, had heart disease, and had survived a colon cancer fortuitously discovered at the time of an operation for diverticulitis. But she had been well enough during the late 1980s to accompany my parents on several of their summer trips to visit my uncle Mark (her son) in France. Pearl had high blood pressure and pretty bad arthritis but was extremely active, driving her own car well into her eighties and traveling to weddings and other family events across the country. She even made the trip to Israel that she and Meyer had begun planning just before he died. In 1991, Pearl and Jessie accompanied my parents to visit Cathy and me in Seattle during my Robert Wood Johnson fellowship. It was not a prescription for relaxation. "There have *never* been two such badly matched traveling companions," my father wrote. "One is hard of hearing and the other doesn't listen so we're constantly repeating and repeating so the two of them are on the same wavelength." Gertie continued to work part-time at a local dry-cleaning store well after she turned eighty.

I vividly remember when Cathy and I would visit Cleveland in the middle and late 1990s with our son, Ben, and, eventually, our daughter, Nina. The three women would sit in the den of my parents' house, reminiscing and bickering. Sharing my father's sense of family history, I recall thinking what a gift it was to have three women born into poverty in Poland in the early twentieth century who were still going strong in the upper-middle-class suburbs of America as the century came to a close. I also loved that I was well into my thirties and still had two grandmothers and a great-aunt doting on me, the first grandchild on both sides of the family. Even better was that they doted on the kids. As a toddler, Ben, in particular, had ample opportunity to interact with his great-grandmothers and Gertie, and he still remembers them well. Ben was "friendly and most solicitous of the older crowd," my father proudly recorded, which was a "blessing."

Jessie was the first to begin to deteriorate. When she fell asleep at ten o'clock on New Year's Eve in 1993, at the age of eighty-six, my mother "wondered, out loud, how many more, if any, New Year's Eves, we'll be together." It was the beginning of a series of premature predictions of Jessie's demise, most of which would be made by my dad. Nevertheless, she had a remarkably large number of ailments, which my father compiled in 1995: worsening blindness and deafness, coughing spasms, stress incontinence, "horrendously itchy" eyes, back pain, hip pain, and chronic diarrhea due to the removal of part of her colon. By the next year, she could not see her great-grandchildren's faces. Meanwhile, she was developing a humped back and had increasing trouble standing up straight. Jessie had also become alarmingly outspoken, showing little or no inclination to censor her thoughts. Over the years, she had heartily criticized my sister Dana's boyfriends, told one of Dana's African American friends that "Black is beautiful!," and once asked me when I was home from college whether I was still a virgin. Such statements and questions always generated considerable laughter, which probably only encouraged her. Even though my mother was the subject of many of Jessie's criticisms, she remained a remarkably dutiful daughter, increasingly putting her life on hold to assist her mother. "I must make note of R.'s extraordinary courage with and devotion for her mother," my father wrote.

Given Jessie's increasing debility, it came as a surprise in 1997 when Pearl, age eighty-eight, died first. Pearl's main medical problems had remained high blood pressure and arthritis. She had also developed what is now called diastolic dysfunction, a condition resulting in a hypertensive patient's lungs filling with fluid if his or her blood pressure gets too high. Over the years, my father had regularly visited Pearl on Sunday mornings for some "venting and gossiping." Pearl was not the warmest person and could be brusque and negative. But she got along well with both my father and his brother, Allan, who also kept close tabs on her. As Pearl's medical problems worsened, my father gradually became more involved, particularly in monitoring Pearl's high blood pressure, which was hard to manage.

I recall being somewhat surprised upon learning of this arrangement. After all, my father was an infectious diseases specialist. Although he was also an internist, it was unlikely that he kept up with recent clinical trials relating to hypertension and heart disease. In contrast, I, as a general internist, dealt with hypertensive patients on a routine basis. On a couple of occasions, I inquired about Pearl's blood pressure and her medications. I recall thinking that if she were my patient, I would have tried for tighter control. I even made a few suggestions about how to treat her, thereby falling into the trap of getting involved in the care of my relatives. But I lived in New York and saw Pearl only on occasion. Plus, she had a history of fainting spells, a possible reason not to lower the blood pressure too much. So I decided to let the subject drop.

Pearl's demise began with a small stroke in mid-December 1997. She was admitted not to the Mount Sinai but to University Hospital, the main hospital of Case Western Reserve. That she had experienced a stroke was particularly relevant, as it was the medical event that she most dreaded. In addition to other friends and family, her sister Shirley had suffered strokes and been incapacitated and miserable for years as a result. Pearl's worst fear, my father wrote, "was to have a stroke and have to live a limited existence, dependent on others for her basic necessities."

It was not clear at first how Pearl would fare. After all, the damage from some strokes is reversible, and this one appeared mild. My father and Allan were near constant presences in the hospital. My dad successfully fed her a meal of juice and Jell-O on December 20, 1997. But Pearl seemed to know that this was the end, talking quietly about Shirley and her husband, Meyer, who had died over twenty years before. And she was right. Shortly after she ate, she suffered a massive bleed in her brain, leaving her comatose. There was no chance of meaningful recovery.

This did not mean that death was imminent. But my father—with his passionate beliefs about limiting suffering at the end of life—thought it should be. Prior to the era of patient autonomy and increased scrutiny of medicine by bioethicists and lawyers, it had been common for physicians to turn up the morphine on patients with massive brain bleeds. I don't remember the exact sequence of events after the bleed nor what my father said at the time, but I had the sense that he had somehow sped things up. He later wrote, somewhat vaguely, that he had been able "to tend to her in her final hours" and "to help her achieve the peaceful end she sought."

Regardless of his involvement, my dad was thrilled—in his own words, "grateful and euphoric"—that Pearl's death at the age of eighty-eight was sudden and without suffering: "I was *happy* Pearl got her wish." He even admitted that he initially had trouble mourning her death because it had gone so well. At the funeral, he had cried only briefly, after seeing some friends from the old Eddy Road neighborhood who reminded him of Pearl "in her prime, in her top form and vibrant, happy, enthusiastic."

In later years, I asked him point-blank what had happened in Pearl's hospital room. He did not remember the specific details, or said he did not, but he admitted that he had guaranteed that she did not linger, making sure that she received enough aggressive medication—presumably morphine—to stop her breathing. This time, it sounded more like euthanasia.

As I had when reading about other end-of-life decisions my father had made, I felt queasy. Do people in comas suffer? In some cases, it appears that they do not. And even if Pearl was suffering, was she suffering enough to warrant such a brazen act as my father—or, at his behest, the hospital staff—may have committed? It seemed hard to justify.

Knowing Pearl as well as I did, I was aware that it was absolutely true that she valued her independence over almost anything. I did not doubt that she was petrified to spend the end of her life either partially paralyzed or bedridden. But when my father wrote that he was glad that Pearl got her wish, it was hard not to think that it was as much his wish as hers. And I was uncomfortable with the fact that he seemed more fixated on *how* she had died rather than *that* she had died. Yes, he had used his skills and power as a physician to help effect a scenario that he, as Pearl's son, believed to be right. I have also recoiled at the prolonged deaths in intensive care units and hospital wards, and I entirely understood his position. The degree to which he had orchestrated the outcome, however, seemed wrong. After all, the cases in which physicians—well meaning or not—had overstepped their bounds were the exact ones that had fostered the growth of bioethics and the adoption of new laws and norms surrounding death and dying.

But I had to ask myself: Could a case be made? My father could argue that he knew the dying arthritis patient as well as anyone and had covered her body with his own when others had been reluctant or afraid to do the right thing. In the case of my grandmother, there was absolutely no doubt that he and his brother knew her best. With death approaching and Pearl experiencing the exact scenario she had so feared, why not move things along? Indeed, once the family members of dying patients are told by doctors that the end is imminent, it is not uncommon for them to become impatient if their loved ones linger. Such sentiments should always give us pause. After all, some relatives' impatience may be due to something other than the desire to end the patient's suffering; for example, they may want to ease their own burdens or obtain inheritances. But if such issues are not in play, is the desire to speed death unreasonable? Hadn't my dad simply taken advantage of his being a physician to accomplish what other loving and grieving children wished they could do?

More subtly, beyond the obligation of not letting his mother linger with an incapacitating stroke, my father was once again motivated by his characteristic need to pay back his relatives for the sacrifices they had made in order for him to become a doctor. If he had the ability to use his medical knowledge to ease his mother's passing, how could he not do it? It was actually his brother, Allan, who conveyed this idea in print, placing an entry into one of my father's journals as Pearl was dying. In it, Allan juxtaposed the nature of her death with what she had meant to him, my father, and the entire family: "My mother is dying her way. She came from a spirit that saved us from the Holocaust by getting us to this country." That is, honoring how Pearl wanted to die was a way of validating the courageous choices she had made during her life.

These same emotions came through in the eulogies that my father and uncle gave for Pearl. She was buried on Cleveland's west side, next to Meyer, near his parents, and surrounded by members of the Jewish social club that had provided cohesion and friendship during her early years in Cleveland. My father was especially pleased that she had an Orthodox funeral and was buried in a traditional shroud, which he knew she would have liked. When religion provided linkages with his family's past, my dad could tolerate, even celebrate, it.

After Pearl's death, my father's and mother's attention naturally shifted back to Jessie. If Pearl had represented a success of modern medicine, living almost ninety mostly healthy years, Jessie embodied the often deleterious consequences of living a long life. By this point, her myriad ailments made it almost impossible for her to leave home, where she now had twenty-four-hour supervision. Either the live-in aide or my mom, who spent enormous amounts of time at Jessie's apartment, had to take her to the bathroom, dress her, and make sure that she ate.

In fact, just before Pearl's death, it had again seemed as if Jessie was about to die. This time, she had developed pneumonia. As had been the case with Pearl, my father had gradually taken over Jessie's medical care from her presumably competent doctors, obviating difficult visits to their offices but raising the same complicated ethical issues. On December 15, 1997, he wrote that "today is probably going to be Jessie's last day." Two days before she had become "confused, upset and terribly agitated." Then she had developed enormous fatigue, sleeping most of the time. My parents, on vigil at Jessie's apartment, had gotten her to eat and drink only a little bit. "I anticipate that without any further improvement in her oral intake," my father wrote in a clinical tone, "that this story is about to conclude."

In anticipation of Jessie's death, he had notified both me and my sister. He also went to the hospital to obtain a death certificate form as well as medication to treat her agitation if necessary. This last maneuver was another reminder of a bygone era. The idea of a physician taking controlled substances from a hospital to use elsewhere would be ludicrous today.

But my father had been wrong. Providing yet another cautionary tale about the folly of caring for one's family members, Jessie once again foiled his considerable prognostic skills. She had woken up the next morning, announced that she was hungry, and eaten a huge breakfast. Within a few days, she was back close to her baseline. She had a staggering number of problems but was not going anywhere. I vividly remember marveling at this turn of events at the time and speaking with her on the phone after her recovery. Was Nana indestructible?

Over the next couple of years, I would see Jessie roughly every four to six months, when I went to Cleveland by myself or with Cathy, Ben, and Nina. The kids, especially Ben, were quite upset at her deterioration. As Jessie could barely see or hear them, she relied on her tactile sense, loving to sit next to them and stroke their hair. Even more remarkable were our phone calls, which required me to practically scream to be heard. Here was a ninety-year-old woman, nearly deaf, blind, weary, and fragile, but she remained utterly sharp, keeping track of the family's doings and, to a lesser extent, world events. My parents briefly contemplated not telling her that Pearl had died, but they realized that she would probably figure it out anyway. Jessie just soldiered on and on.

To what degree was she suffering? At one point, my father termed her life a "most unhappy existence." It was certainly one that he himself did not see as worth living. Yet despite being "emotionally quite unhappy" at all of her medical woes, Jessie never indicated in any manner that she was ready to give up or that she wanted to die. Her tenacity, we suspected, stemmed in large part from her continued desire to try, from her apartment couch, to provide profuse advice to the rest of us about how to live our lives. Her involvement was excessive, to be sure, but it was also inspiring that she still cared so very much.

My father was extremely concerned with the effect that Jessie's ongoing infirmity was having on my mother, who spent large amounts of time at the apartment and took each new medical or psychological downturn very hard. "Ronnie is at the end of her patience, emotionally and even physically, and I fear for her well-being during this continuing ordeal," he remarked in 1996. "She is her nurse and her only link with the outside world." Even after they hired a full-time aide to help Jessie, my parents were reluctant to spend much time away. Although my sister and I insisted that they go on a special vacation for their fortieth wedding anniversary, in November 1998, they just stayed in Cleveland. In his journal entry for that day, my father wrote that "Jessie's condition throttles Ronnie's and my lives, as we cannot shed the responsibility for her care and comfort." This was their choice, but they were not without some regret. "We must make a greater effort to try and live a more normal life divorced as much as possible from the inevitable deterioration of our elderly parents and aunt," my dad wrote in 1996. But they never did.

As my father contemplated what would eventually happen to Jessie, his touchstone was again the 1996 case of the patient with severe arthritis and vascular disease. There were, of course, substantial differences—most notably, that Jessie was not yet end stage and was not hospitalized. He noted that were Jessie to be hospitalized, she would surely have a do-not-resuscitate order, unlike the earlier patient. But he wanted to keep her out of the hospital entirely. "The question really comes down to whether or not I can orchestrate and carry out her dying at home," my dad wrote. "Once she goes into the hospital, I lose my ability to impact the *total* decision-making process."

Jessie made it until February 2000, more than two years after Pearl's death. At that point, she was ninety-three years old. What happened first was worsening shortness of breath and agitation. My father, sticking to his plan, initially tried to manage her symptoms in the apartment by giving her sedatives. Fortunately, he quickly realized that he was in over his head. By this point, my father had left the Mount Sinai and had no admitting privileges, even if he had wanted to be on record as his mother-in-law's doctor. He called Jessie's old internist, who agreed to admit her, although this doctor was going on vacation the next day.

Once the admission testing was done, her medical condition became clearer. Apparently she had suffered one or more heart attacks and had gone into congestive heart failure. The fluid in her lungs was making her short of breath.

I remember having a series of uncomfortable phone calls with my father at this point. Again, he seemed to be too involved, running the case instead of relying on the judgment of Jessie's actual doctors. But I, too, was drawn to the medical details. From where I stood, it seemed as if Jessie had a treatable condition. Mind you, I did not mean anything invasive. But I speculated that giving her diuretics and other pills to treat her heart failure would be reasonable and might be a way for her to go back home.

My father, however, was pushing hard in the other direction, desperately seeking to avoid "meaningless treatments that wouldn't change the ultimate outcome." He saw her deteriorating heart function as the final straw, thinking that it should be viewed not as reversible but as a mechanism for easing Jessie into death. This thinking reminded me of the designation of pneumonia as the old man's friend in the days before antibiotics. Everyone had to die of something, both then and now, and, in this case, my dad thought Jessie's heart should be the cause. I knew this decision was based on his thoughtful assessment of both Jessie's medical condition and its effects on those around her, although I did not understand it exactly until I later read his journal entries. Plus, I was five hundred miles away and not involved in my grandmother's day-to-day care. I essentially deferred to my father, although I remained upset at the situation. Indeed, my dad was so intent on orchestrating Jessie's death that he had booked a funeral home for later in the week and was urging my sister, me, and other relatives to clear our calendars.

But there were two major problems. First, my father's urgent pleas for the medical staff to aggressively administer morphine—which treats some aspects of congestive heart failure but can also cause patients to stop breathing—were met with resistance. Four years earlier, he had marched down the wards of this hospital doing whatever he wanted with impunity, even physically preventing CPR. But now, everything had changed. As he later wrote, "My problem with the staff . . . was getting enough morphine into Nana to ease her passing." Her "quick final exit" became stalled "when the staff rebelled at my pushing the dose of morphine." On at least one occasion, it seems, the nurses lowered the rate of the morphine drip as my father was sleeping in the room. What apparently did not occur—but probably would have at my hospital, the Columbia campus of New York–Presbyterian Hospital—was someone calling for an urgent ethics consult to mediate between my father's demands and the reluctance of Jessie's physicians and nurses to follow his wishes.

Second, Jessie was rallying. Once again, my father had to eat his words. "As it turns out, my accuracy at predicting Nana's passing suffered yet another setback today," he admitted, "as she suddenly began to breathe more normally than I would have thought possible." This time, however, even Jessie had had enough. On the afternoon of February 6, 2000, five days after she entered the hospital, she finally stopped breathing.

The graveside funeral was a small one, mostly close relatives. Having spent most of her life elsewhere, Jessie had few friends in Cleveland. My father, my sister, and I spoke; our eulogies were celebrations of her life, replete with anecdotes about her strong opinions and loose tongue. But even more so than with Pearl, who had suffered a major, irreversible medical event, I remained uncomfortable with my father's seemingly unilateral decision to withhold certain treatments and thus speed Jessie's death. My sister, Dana, was actually surprised that Jessie had not lived at least until the birth of her first child, Gianna, in the summer of 2000. Despite her major infirmities, Jessie had been ardently awaiting this event. It seemed to me that there was a reasonable chance that with more aggressive treatment of the heart failure, Jessie might actually have reached this goal. And even though the pre-death planning had made it easier for me to attend the funeral and mourn with my family, it struck me as inappropriate to try to time someone's death in this manner.

So how did my father, as revealed in his writings, build a case for what he had tried to accomplish? First, he emphasized Jessie's miserable quality of life. Even if she still derived a degree of pleasure from eating and hearing about her loved ones, she was constantly unhappy, suffering from—and complaining about—one or more of her countless worsening maladies. My father seemed to have concluded that no one that miserable could genuinely want to undergo aggressive measures that would perpetuate such a state.

Second, my dad cited the toll Jessie's poor health was taking on my mom, whose endurance, after years of immersion in Jessie's care, was waning, raising the possibility that she might experience some type of physical or emotional breakdown. "It was time!" he wrote. "We could have kept her going for a few more days or perhaps even a couple of weeks, but the physical costs to her and the emotional cost to R would have been horrible! Absolutely, utterly HORRIBLE." Plus, my parents' slavish devotion to Jessie was, my father wrote, having a negative impact on their "relations with our kids and grandchildren." That is, my parents' choosing to stay in Cleveland meant fewer trips to New York and missing family events, which my sister, Dana, in particular, found objectionable. After Jessie died, my father wrote: "R and I can also now *reclaim* our lives together, to travel together, to plan excursions."

As someone working in bioethics, with its emphasis on the rights of patients, I was alarmed to see my father invoke such considerations when making decisions about how long someone was entitled to live. I have little doubt that the fantasy ethics consultant that I imagined would have told my father to back off and rebuked him for conflating the goal of making Jessie comfortable as she died with that of trying to hasten her death. The bioethicist would have worked hard to elicit Jessie's opinion as well as that of my mother, her nearest relative and primary caregiver. The Columbia ethics committee on which I sat for twenty years had at times encountered similar cases, in which paternalistic doctors—who were sure that they knew best—tried to exclude patients and family members from life-and-death decisions. My colleagues and I nearly always rejected such actions. What made my father's behavior especially outrageous in this instance was his highly unorthodox decision to include my mother's emotional well-being as part of his calculus when weighing Jessie's various therapeutic options.

But there was another way to view this complicated dynamic between a dying woman and her loving family. If Jessie had briefly regained her eyesight, hearing, and other faculties and realized what her condition was doing to her beloved daughter, would she have actually agreed with my dad? It is impossible to know, but if, as in the aphorism that "a physician's job is to relieve often and comfort always," it might be argued that there was no one but my father who had the medical skills, emotional insight, and familial allegiance to make the choices in question. It might also be argued, more provocatively, that the full-on embrace of patient autonomy by my generation of bioethicists precluded us from even considering that my father's highly paternalistic actions in Jessie's—or Pearl's—death might have been justified. A few weeks before Jessie died, my dad had made one of his countless visits to her apartment and found her to be "less communicative," possibly indicative of even more deterioration. As he gave her his customary kiss good-bye on her forehead, he had made her a promise: she "would not suffer at all when the time came." Armed with as much morphine as he could round up from the resistant nursing staff, he kept his word.

Six days after Jessie's death, my father recorded his final thoughts on what had happened and had no regrets. Once again referencing the misuse of technology that he had seen at the end of life, he was pleased to have spared Jessie any "slippery slope madness." He added that he and his brother had done the same for Pearl two years before. Then, vividly linking the filial and professional roles he had chosen in life, he concluded with a triumphant thrust: "So both mothers were spared suffering at the ends of their lives because their 'sons' were doctors who 'acted.'" One might argue that what had transpired crossed a dangerous line, but this was surely an inspiring image of what a physician—in this case, a loving physician—could achieve.

Of course, my father well knew that this type of doctor-driven paternalism was not the ultimate answer to improving medical decision-making. So when it came to my dad's managing the medical care of the third old lady, his aunt Gertie, she was a more active participant. To some degree, this choice reflected Gertie's personality. In contrast to Jessie, Gertie had responded to her increasing infirmities by articulating limits to future possible treatments.

By the fall of 2000, Gertie was ninety-one years old and had moved into a nursing home. My father and Allan visited her regularly, often bringing her a corned-beef sandwich, which reminded her of the good old days. I saw Gertie for the last time that December. Although extremely frail, she was thrilled to see me and Cathy, as well as Ben and Nina, whom we brought along.

By February 2001, however, Gertie was "dwindling away," eating and drinking less. My father wrote that she was "adamant" about not returning to the hospital when she worsened. Of course, he fully concurred. Then, on March 21, coincidentally the birthday of her brother Mickey, she died. "While waiting in the dining room for lunch," my father movingly wrote, "my Aunt Gertie put her head down on the table and left us, as peacefully and calmly as we had hoped." It was the sort of death that almost everyone—from paternalistic physicians like my dad to people trained in autonomy-based bioethics like myself—hoped for.

Still, it was tough for my father. "Gertie's passing will be a blessing for her," he wrote a month before her death, "but I'll be saddened, as she is the last living link with my father's family and that generation."

My dad would remain immersed in the medical illnesses of other relatives and friends, but the end-of-life care of Pearl, Jessie, and Gertie represented what he might have termed one of his final official duties as both a son and a physician. Plus, my father's world was shaking, both figuratively and literally. His beloved Mount Sinai Hospital was in turmoil, forcing him to take early retirement. And the disease that would come to dominate the rest of his life—Parkinson's—was beginning to rear its head.

CHAPTER EIGHT

Growing Disillusionment

My father and I practiced medicine concurrently for a dozen years, from 1986 to 1998. Unfortunately, this period—especially the later years—was my father's least happy time as a physician. Beset by demands from insurance companies, dealing with increasing amounts of paperwork and a hospital that was suffering financially, he realized that the career he had fashioned as a consultant, teacher, and researcher was becoming much less viable. Even worse, he could not hide his frustration and contempt for what was happening, which led him to spoil his thirty-fifth medical school reunion with a rant.

I, on the other hand, was just beginning my career in the late 1980s and early 1990s, first as a house officer and then as an assistant professor. I experienced many of the same frustrations but, perhaps due to lower expectations and the enthusiasm of youth, did not wear my annoyance on my sleeve. Having so admired my father as a physician, I found it painful to see him so unhappy and, frankly, to listen to his tirades. His journals, not surprisingly, chronicle the many ways in which medicine—which had once brought him such joy—now did the opposite. Although he tried to channel his energies into specific projects, most notably what he called a manifesto on the inappropriate use of antibiotics, most of them never came to fruition.

Meanwhile, drawing on my training in history and bioethics and on what I had learned from my father during the prime of his career, I tried to practice a patient-centered form of medicine that fit within the new realities of managed care, time constraints, and the need to see medicine as a part of one's larger life—something my father was never really able to do.

To my dad's credit, at some point he realized that he was becoming too negative. While staying with my uncle Mark in the summer of 1987 and during several subsequent visits to France, he made a point of "smelling the roses," acknowledging moments that he called the "perfect instants of our lives." On at least one occasion, he reported having experienced "total and entire relaxation." His parents had been born into poverty in Poland, and he into a working-class home in East Cleveland, yet here he was, lounging on the terrace of a villa in the south of France. My dad was a respected physician married to a wonderful woman who was his "compass," and he was the father of two successful children. The three old ladies were doing well at that time, and Jessie, also born in Poland, was healthy enough to come to France each summer. "These are the 'good old days' I'll fondly remember tomorrow," he wrote in 1989, "and things will never be less complicated than they are just now."

Still, he admitted, he was too often guilty of "letting the little things, the glitches and annoyances" become the "dominant facts" of his life. That my father kept journals was probably a blessing in this regard. Amid the chronicling of his relatives' medical problems and the milestones of his children and grandchildren are repetitive, angry entries about the decline of both his revered Mount Sinai Hospital and the medical system in general. My mother, my sister, and I got earfuls of this, but his journals got even more.

Just what was bothering my father so much? Some of it was his frustration about being asked to juggle antibiotics in patients who deserved to be left alone, but there were deeper problems. One of the first about which he wrote with regularity was an issue within the medical profession itself. Having trained to be a physician who compulsively checked every laboratory value and physical finding of his patients, my dad was growing irritated at specialists and sub-specialists who saw their role as diagnosing and fixing very narrow problems—such as clogged arteries or thinning bones—without, apparently, any interest in the overall medical and emotional lives of the patients who had these conditions. "I have become increasingly dismayed," he wrote in 1984, "by the frustrations of trying to practice and promote the *proper* execution of medicine, my chosen life's endeavor."

In one journal entry, my father divided what he perceived as unsatisfactory physicians into three groups. First were the automatons, who were not necessarily bad doctors but who lacked passion for their work. Second were the opportunists, who expected and demanded enormous financial rewards for their efforts. The third group—by far the worst—were the "outright charlatans, a mixture of idiots, thieves, incompetents and general misfits whom our system fails to screen out of the educational process and our profession hasn't the guts to eliminate from their protected position in the establishment."

My father directly pointed fingers: certain orthopedists, gynecologists, and urologists were among the worst offenders. He reported seeing the same mistakes over and over "because no one is paying attention to the patient as a total organism, rather than a bone or a joint or a uterus or a kidney or a bladder." By no means did he mean to indict all practitioners in these fields. The guilty doctors were "fortunately a minority." But when physicians did not care about basic concepts they had learned about in medical school—fluid balance, the body's healing processes, and the balance between disease-causing bacteria and normal flora—they became "tunnel-vision technicians." In April 1984, my father wrote a letter full of these types of complaints to his dear friend James J. Rahal, a New York infectious diseases specialist who had also trained with Louis Weinstein. "I'm tired of these young whipper-snappers who know only how to perform 'oscopies' and other procedures, but haven't the slightest idea of what practicing medicine really means," he said. "I'm tired of the rude and stupid physicians who don't understand the basic courtesy involved in a consultation, who think nothing of frantically asking you to drop everything to bail them out and then never get back to you after you do so." In a reply, Rahal supportively termed the missive the "lament of a committed physician," but he seemed to be taken aback at my father's anger.

Another group of physicians that at times disappointed my dad were family physicians. At first glance, one might think this surprising, given the specialty's emphasis on comprehensive care of patients and their families, but my father had encountered several such colleagues who he believed were lacking. In one instance, he found himself being the first doctor to address the emotional concerns of a patient with Crohn's disease who was going to need surgery and an ileostomy (an opening in the abdomen for expelling intestinal waste). That a specialist, and not the woman's family physician, was the one actually caring for the whole patient was unsatisfactory.

My father's gripe with family physicians raised hackles within our own family. My wife's dad, Sam Seibel, was a highly competent general practitioner on Long Island for decades. When he first met my dad, he was planning to take board examinations in family medicine, the specialty that had come to encompass the broad sort of medicine that he practiced. At that Sunday brunch, my dad could not resist saying how often he had to repair the damage that certain family physicians had caused. Sam, although not yet boarded in the field, was understandably a little defensive. The ensuing discussion, which grew heated for a while, led my sister to joke that the two doctors needed to go outside and settle matters with a duel.

I was embarrassed by both the vehemence of my father's complaints and the particular venue in which he had chosen to make them known. Even if he did not mean to imply that he and his colleagues were superior to physicians in the specialty of my soon-to-be father-in-law, his comments struck me as haughty. In addition, he was painting with far too broad a brush, condemning entire groups of physicians for the sins of a few, something that he at least recognized he might be doing when writing in his journals. I asked him to tone it down when we were with Sam, which he agreed to do. But his profound disappointment with the efforts of certain physicians remained on his front burner. Like Robert Loeb and many other great professors, my dad simply could not stomach physicians who did not "give it their all" and thus cut corners on patient care.

Also in my father's line of fire were "the increasing number of house officers who appear not to understand the rare privilege they have been given, to become physicians." Of course, it was not all their fault. Thanks in large part to the Libby Zion case, training programs had finally begun to cut residents' work hours. To some degree, I had benefited from this new approach. Not surprisingly, my father and many physicians from his generation were wary of what would become characterized as shift work. If 24/7 immersion in patient care was the gold standard, even an eighty-hour-maximum workweek—the first reduction that was widely implemented— seemed deleterious for both learning medicine and attending to patients. Young physicians increasingly wanted to "get home in time for whatever" and "not be burdened with concerns about what he/ she left behind," my father derisively wrote. "Someone else is covering—I don't have to worry!"

But my dad was even angrier at the bureaucracy that had come to dominate medicine. Beginning in the 1980s and increasing over time, it was no longer adequate for physicians to examine patients and leave their findings and recommendations in the medical charts. Rather, it was necessary to leave certain types of notes, ones that did not necessarily convey useful medical information but contained details that satisfied regulatory agencies or ensured that the hospital got appropriately paid for its services. "My daily activities in the hospital are already swinging drastically in favor of documenting rather than doing," my father wrote in 1992. "I am a cog in a large, impersonal juggernaut of activity, much of it wasteful."

What especially irked him was the fact that the requests for greater documentation came from "non-professional data gatherers" and "management maniacs" who could call into question "the activities of a physician trying to care for an evolving biological process." For example, Medicare was constantly changing its coding system, leading to errors and interfering with the reimbursements for my father's consultations. He saw all of these changes as direct threats to both the authority of physicians and the art of medicine. Future doctors, he feared, would not use their own experience and judgment but would merely carry out diagnostic and treatment protocols designed by managers and insurers. My dad was too ill by 2007 to read Jerome Groopman's book *How Doctors Think*, but he would have agreed with Groopman's concern that reliance on generic patient profiles leads modern doctors to "ignore the individual characteristics of the patient."

Related to the growing bureaucratization of medicine were changes in medical education. The notion of being a specialist in infectious diseases and yet not doing one's own Gram stains was anathema to my father. One of his "Ten Commandments in Infectious Diseases," which he distributed annually to his students, was "Thou shalt have no other Gods before the Gram stain." Being directly involved in the process by which a particular infectious organism was identified was a "connection to the world of microbiology," the best way for a specialist to make an accurate diagnosis and then recommend an effective therapy. Moreover, senior physicians had a duty to teach their junior colleagues and medical students how to do Gram stains, examine urine specimens under the microscope, and spin their patients' blood in a centrifuge to check for anemia—as I had done during my medical school rotations and as a house officer.

But now this type of intimate knowledge was being threatened. As medical documentation became more formalized, with accreditations necessary for hospital laboratories and other facilities, the information obtained in makeshift resident labs could no longer be considered official. Cleveland's University Hospital, the main teaching center for Case Western Reserve medical students, attempted to solve this problem by renaming them teaching labs, used to train students but not for patient care. Unfortunately, when asked by an inspector from the Joint Commission on Accreditation for Hospitals whether the information he was obtaining in the laboratory would be used in patient care, a Case medical student—telling the truth—said yes. The dean of the medical school closed the labs the next day.

It was a similar story in other teaching hospitals, including Columbia-Presbyterian. Not only medical students but all the physicians in the hospital became more and more dependent on information generated by other hospital staff members, such as laboratory technicians and radiologists. Reading a report on a piece of paper or a computer screen had replaced looking at actual specimens. This development was especially difficult for my father and his generation, who prided themselves on seeing everything with their own eyes, whether it was a deteriorating patient in the middle of the night or that patient's phlegm, urine, or blood. Now the nurses paged whatever doctor was covering, and that doctor just read the reports in patient's record. As late as 1995, my father was still teaching medical students how to do Gram stains, running what was probably one of the last such educational efforts in the country. That same year he learned that Mount Sinai Hospital was planning to move its *actual* microbiology laboratory off-campus, meaning that the few remaining doctors who still did their own smears or reviewed those prepared by the laboratory would not even be able to do that. Predictably, he termed this action "insanity."

Other paperwork was "drowning" my father as well: "letters, memos, forms, claims, licenses, applications." To order certain tests or examinations, one had to obtain permission or prior approval from insurance companies, which my father believed were "taking over the profession" by promoting "cookbook medicine." Third-party payers, who did not begin to understand the complicated cases they were evaluating, were "passing judgment *from a distance* on proper medical care." My father tried to get his secretary to handle these matters, but he often had to write letters or make phone calls. Given his frustration with the middlemen who he felt were interfering with the practice of medicine and raising costs, he wanted physicians themselves "to develop and monitor treatment guidelines for our new healthcare system." My dad also became an advocate for a single-payer model and was disappointed at the failure of the Clinton administration to reform health care in 1994.

But my father did not just sit around and complain. Far from it. He was heavily involved in trying to help the Mount Sinai deal with all of the new requirements and was constantly giving what he termed "respected and even well-received" feedback to members of the hospital's hierarchy. Toward the end of 1992, for example, the Mount Sinai computerized its laboratory system as a way to improve

accountability and accuracy. But what resulted were enormous printouts of laboratory data, as much as two hundred pages per patient,
which were dutifully inserted into the medical charts. Realizing that
information generated in such a format was not only unwieldy but
probably confusing, my father went to the pathologist who ran the
laboratory system to alert him about the problem. The pathologist
referred him to the hospital's computer information specialist, who
agreed to contact the company in charge of the project to correct
the glitch. Apparently, my father had been the only person to reg-
ister a complaint. The episode, he later wrote, "clearly illustrates a
total, I mean absolutely, complete lack of quality-control supervision
of the laboratory."

Seeing the opportunity for meaningful change, my dad used this
episode to urge the formation of a committee of physicians and staff
members to computerize the storage and retrieval of patient data "in
an organized and a visionary fashion." But after one "very enthusiastic opening meeting," my father learned that two of the most essential committee members, the computer specialist and the nursing
administrator, were probably going to be let go, essentially dooming
the committee. "To say that this is pulling out the rug from under
me is no exaggeration," he wrote.

And on it went, as Dr. Phillip Lerner and a small band of fellow
physician-reformers tried to influence the inevitable transforma-
tions at the Mount Sinai. Their efforts were largely ineffective. At
times, my father wondered why he was even bothering. "Why am I
so stubbornly pursuing this when no one else seems concerned—at
all concerned?" he asked himself after the incident with the excessive
printouts. The answer, for him, was always the same. "The bottom
line is patient care," he wrote. "If it is being compromised by this
inanity, I simply can't abide it in any way, shape or form." It was, as
James Rahal had said, the lament of a committed physician.

It was this devotion to the patient, which he had first embraced
so passionately at the Western Reserve School of Medicine in the
1950s, that led to my father's unfortunate misstep at his thirty-
fifth medical school reunion in 1993. After dinner, a number of his
classmates stood up to speak, all discussing their careers, families,

and adventures since the last reunion. A few spoke more substantively about health-care reform and other changes in medicine. But my father, probably assuming that he was preaching to the choir, launched into a tirade about how his professional life had been shattered. He did not write down his exact remarks that night but it is reasonable to assume they resembled what he had been recording in his journals: anger at the insurance companies, anger at his hospital's administrators, and possibly even anger at certain clinical specialties, representatives of which may have been in the audience. When I first heard this story, I thought of the 1959 film *The Last Angry Man*, which I watched with my dad when I was a teenager. In the movie, Paul Muni plays a revered physician who devotes his life to caring for a poor, immigrant community but who gets unhinged by the business tactics of his younger competitors and the social changes in his neighborhood. At that point, my father had not yet soured on medicine, but I recall his fierce identification with the Muni character.

He did record in his journals the reaction of his fellow classmates to his reunion diatribe: "stony silence." To make matters worse, when he sat down, my mother rightly upbraided him for not mentioning her at all when his other classmates had made a point of thanking their spouses. He deeply regretted his actions, especially snubbing my mother—"my oxygen, my anchor"—and realized how "preoccupied and disturbed this has all made me, influencing my behavior almost in an uncontrollable way." He was "obsessed" with the topic and perhaps even "unstable."

Having frequently heard my father's gripes and having been told about the reunion debacle, I was not surprised by much of what I read in his journals from these years. But it was profoundly sad for me to see him questioning his own sanity, something that he did only privately. It was these entries that led me to think of my father's old hero Ignaz Semmelweis, the physician who made the brilliant discovery about the transmission of puerperal fever via unwashed hands but who later grew fanatical about the subject and died in a mental institution. Fortunately, my dad's condition—which he termed, at various times, an agitated depression, an anxiety disorder, or panic attacks—never reached that point. But the obsessive nature of the two quests was not dissimilar. After the reunion, my father pledged to "shed this yoke, as it is threatening to get out of hand and literally consume me."

He never really did. Activities that once had generated pleasure, such as running the infectious diseases teaching committee for medical students, no longer made him happy. Curriculum changes at the medical school were "window dressing" that avoided the main problem: "Where have all the good teachers gone?" Even worse was that attendance for the committee, still given during the spring of the second year of medical school, had dropped dramatically as students increasingly chose instead to study for their upcoming national board examinations. In 1995, for example, only about forty students (one-quarter of the class) attended with some regularity, despite the fact that my father and his colleagues dutifully rewrote the syllabus every year and made sure to deliver interesting lectures. "Will have to explore other options for next year," he concluded with resignation. Three years later, things were no better: "Few showed up for the sessions."

Even more remarkable, in some ways, was my dad's loss of enthusiasm for writing and scholarship. Even though he had rejected a traditional academic pathway when he left Boston, he had been remarkably productive in generating case studies, book chapters, and other manuscripts during his years in Cleveland—work that gave him "some cachet in the ID community." I knew he was proud of these writings because he presented me with a collection of his reprints at some point during my medical school or residency training. I recall sharing them with my Columbia colleagues on several occasions when we had a relevant case.

By the mid-1990s, however, his output had slowed to a trickle. Some of this was natural, perhaps, as he had reached his sixties, and his responsibilities had, if anything, increased: "There is always another paper to write, a chapter to revise, a lecture to update, a seminar to organize." But the same ennui that affected his clinical work and teaching had spread to his scholarship. For example, he turned in a review article on nocardiosis, a lung infection in which he was an expert, months late. He correctly predicted that it would be his last review article, as he had "lost [his] enthusiasm for such undertakings as well as the freedom to allocate my time to undertake such projects." I now know that part of what he was doing, ironically, was compulsively writing in his journals about his inability to write.

As early as 1987, my father had begun musing about authoring a paper that summarized his "maverick viewpoints about antibiotic therapy." Louis Weinstein, Max Finland, and many of the other founding fathers of infectious diseases had quickly realized that the new wonder drugs could be used improperly, leading to bacterial resistance and other unfortunate outcomes. My dad had been an apostle of this viewpoint throughout his career, insisting particularly that diagnostic imprecision had led to rampant misuse of antibiotics, even by specialists in the field. Over the years, he had developed other counterintuitive beliefs about antibiotics, which he had taught in the classroom and on the wards. One major point that my father consistently emphasized was that—counter to common opinion—antibiotics do not cure infections. Rather, they assist the body's host defenses in doing so. Not appreciating this, clinicians often gave antibiotics for too long and at doses that were too high, which did more harm than good, including promoting the growth of resistant bacteria. "Why," he liked to ask his colleagues, "do we not study precisely how much antibiotic is needed in a given situation and then give no more?" Sometimes only "very small doses" may be necessary to turn the tide. Another of my dad's mottos was "Give a first-generation antibiotic for a first-generation infection," again underscoring how doctors tended to overuse newer, more expensive antibiotics, assuming they were necessarily better. One of the forces encouraging this misguided approach was the pharmaceutical industry, which was engaged in what he called an "almost mindless, frantic search for and deluge of ever more potent agents," rather than studying the advantages and pitfalls of existing antibiotics.

By ignoring what Louis Pasteur had termed the terrain and focusing too closely on the germ, medicine had missed an opportunity to study and improve how patients' immunological systems responded to infections. "The Forgotten Host" was the title of an article by bacteriologist Ernest Jawetz from the May 1955 of the *Stanford Medical Bulletin* that my father had dug up on this topic. Physicians now placed too much focus on specific bacteria that grew from cultures of bodily fluids. Many of these were merely colonizers, present but not causing actual disease. Meanwhile, drug-resistant bacteria—reflexively termed *killer bugs* or *superbugs*—actually grew normally or sluggishly in patients with intact immune systems. My father even put forth the somewhat heretical opinion that nosocomial infections—infections that patients acquired in the hospital and that were the source of enormous consternation among administrators and regulatory agencies—often caused little actual harm.

My dad approached a friend, the editor of a major infectious diseases journal, who indicated interest in an article that made these points. The piece would be my father's "main academic contribution to infectious diseases." I recall him mentioning his proposed "antibiotic polemic" to me on many occasions. At some point, I began actively urging him to finish it. But, although he wrote several one- or two-page outlines in his journals, he never did.

His inability to finish this project, plus the continuing travails at the Mount Sinai, plus what was probably a degree of mental illness led him to muse frequently in his journals about his legacy. He often found himself wanting. At one meeting of the Infectious Diseases Society of America, he compared his "meager achievements" to those of several peers being given lifetime achievement awards. Due to his career choices, a lack of ego, and an unwillingness to seek recognition, he had chosen instead to be more of a "foot soldier." On another occasion, a visit by a renowned infectious diseases specialist from Tufts, his former institution, reminded my father "what I might have become had I elected to remain in Boston, as Dr. Weinstein implored me to do."

At some point, my dad began collecting quotations that reflected his mood. He approvingly cited the writer Mary McCarthy, who once said, "The belief in progress that animated my youth has vanished." Elsewhere, he quoted an anonymous source as saying, "A man has only so many years of optimism." He also increasingly contemplated his own mortality. In one's forties and fifties, he wrote in 1994 at the age of sixty-one, "there's lots of time left." But in your sixties and early seventies, with contemporaries dying, "that means 5 or 10 or 15 years is what's left." On the fiftieth anniversary of D-day, June 6, 1994, he called himself "old enough to have experienced history." On another occasion, when visiting his father's and grandparents' graves at the cemetery that housed members of my family's old Jewish club, he ran into an acquaintance from the old Glenville neighborhood. "Seeing him there was a bit jarring," my father wrote, "since he looks so much like his mother and he's now an old man and, by some measures, I guess so am I." In the summer of 1997, on the way to Cape Cod, we stopped to visit Louis Weinstein, my dad's old mentor, at his home in Newton, Massachusetts. Weinstein was eighty-nine years old and in declining health, but my father was glad to see him and thanked him one last time for giving him such a great opportunity. By this point, my dad had begun to muse about an early retirement, something that would have seemed inconceivable a few years earlier.

Amid this profound negativity, my father experienced many happy events during these years, which he dutifully recorded in his journals as well. In 1990, he received a major teaching award from the medical school. As his own severest critic, he wrote that he did not need to hear from others that he was doing a good job, but he admitted that the award was "long overdue." The next year, the editors of the prestigious *Harrison's Principles of Internal Medicine* asked him to write a chapter on actinomycosis, a fungal infection on which he was a recognized expert. Writing for this particular textbook was something he had actually dreamed about doing since medical school. And, in September 1993, he finally hired an associate to help him cover the large number of infectious diseases consultations he received and ideally free up his time for teaching and research. The fact that the associate was a woman, Cindy Gustaferro, showed how much medicine had changed since my dad went to medical school.

Her gender mattered little to him; he just wanted a partner who would be as obsessive as he was.

Gustaferro's appearance was especially notable for another reason. "I'm not on call this weekend!" my father wrote on September 26. "The very first time in 20 years I don't have to think about the hospital at all!" Being on call for twenty years did not mean that my father constantly got bothered every weeknight and weekend, but when there was a crisis, he surely did, and at times he headed back to the hospital. As someone whose sanity depends on patient-free vacations and catching up on sleep over the weekend, I can only shudder at the notion of being on call for over seven thousand straight days.

But my father's greatest joys during the 1990s were surely my and my sister's marriages, followed by the birth of his grandchildren. My wedding to Cathy was in Brooklyn in August 1990 and my father was especially happy that it—at least temporarily—reunited the family that had scattered within and beyond Cleveland. As usual, his emotions were less apparent in public than they were in his journals, where he wrote, "I was literally bursting with happiness, especially with all the family and friends around to share it with me." Remarkably, four parents and four grandparents (Jessie, Pearl, and Cathy's grandparents Teddy and Norma) plus Aunt Gertie were present. As usual, my father took note of who was not there, especially feeling the absence of his dad, Meyer.

Best of all, the wedding, at least transiently, distracted my father's attention from the "turmoil" of the hospital. Anyone reading his description of the wedding, he wryly noted, would "notice a rather different mood in the writer." The wedding gave him "new impetus to re-evaluate and carry on."

Even more momentous, however, was the birth of Cathy's and my first child, Ben, on January 20, 1993. At this point, we were living in Seattle and I was completing my fellowship. Within twelve hours of Ben's birth, my father had begun another journal, inscribed "To my grandson, Ben Michael Lerner." Ben was born on the day of Bill Clinton's first inauguration but my father had no trouble terming his birth "the most eventful happening of the day," especially because he was the first member of the next generation of his family. That Ben was named after Phil's beloved grandfather Ben Lerner as well as his father and father-in-law (Michael was a tribute to Meyer and Mannie) ensured that there would be a family-history lesson in the inaugural entry of the new journal: the first Ben Lerner's courageous decision to leave Poland, Meyer's leaving school early and toiling as a furrier, and my father's own fortunate pathway into medicine. Meyer and Mannie, he wrote, "would have savored this moment even more passionately than I." Two years later, when Cathy and I were back in New York, our daughter, Nina, was born. "Welcome dear one to my heart and our family," my father wrote, beginning a series of journal entries to Nina to accompany those that he continued to write to Ben.

Another source of joy for my dad was my evolving medical career. Yes, we disagreed about how to balance paternalism and autonomy, and the changes in medicine complicated my career path, but I had followed my father into academic medicine. Like him, I eschewed a traditional private practice, instead seeing clinic patients part of the time, teaching medical students and residents, and doing research. As with many, if not most, physicians I encountered, my father did not quite understand the idea of a research career in the history of medicine. Most researchers worked in laboratories or studied the medical outcomes of living patients, as he had. But he (and my mother) could not have been more enthusiastic, especially since I was doing what I loved. My dad had once known this same type of exhilaration.

I was amused, therefore, when I read what he had recorded in a journal entry in January 1996 when he was visiting us in New York. After having dinner on a Saturday night, I had apparently sat down to do work, looked at my father, and said good-naturedly, "It's your fault." "I suppose it is," he wrote. Yes, the apple had not fallen far from the tree. But another journal entry, this one from November 1998, around the time of the publication of my first book, surprised me. "I think (in fact, I know)," my father wrote to me, "that you are more ambitious and far more disciplined than I ever was." Having grown up thinking of my dad as the most disciplined person that I knew—and myself as insufficiently disciplined—it was hard to read these words. But it helped to explain his inability, at least later in life, to complete the projects that he knew he should.

I readily used my father's expertise when I began to write articles on the history of medicine for both medical and historical journals. He was especially helpful when I researched infectious diseases, as he had personally encountered some of the events I described, but he was even more valuable as an editor, cutting down my expansive language into acceptable nuggets. He also relished inviting me to Cleveland to give talks, as my being there with my family had the added advantage of allowing him to see his grandchildren. I must admit that I loved these gigs, as I got to lecture in front of relatives, friends, and doctors I had known for years. It was also great seeing how proud these appearances made my father (and mother).

One particularly memorable visit was in October 1997, just before my dad's sixty-fifth birthday, when I spoke on the history of breast cancer at the Allen Memorial Library. The night before, my father and I had suffered together as our cursed Cleveland Indians lost game seven of the World Series to the Florida Marlins after leading the game going into the bottom of the ninth inning.

During these years, my father and I worked hard on being more emotional with each other. He had never been one to display his emotions outwardly and I, his doctor son, was a chip off the old block. But now, when I left Cleveland to return home or when he departed from New York, we hugged and made sure to say "I love you." Later on, when I read my father's accounts of these episodes, I realized how hard it could be for him to display his profound feelings so openly. "It's a bit difficult with a son, this hugging business," he wrote in 1994, "to be careful and not overdo it with your grown man."

During these visits, my dad's discontent with medicine inevitably came up. I did my best to let him vent. In some ways, however, I disagreed with what he so passionately believed. Doctors of my generation entered the profession using different approaches. For example, I was much less willing to use my clinical judgment alone to make decisions for my patients. Among medical specialties, general internal medicine, which I practiced, had particularly embraced the notion of evidence-based medicine, which relied on sophisticated clinical trials and meta-analyses to ascertain the value of screening procedures and therapies. As a historian, I was well aware of how value laden and nonobjective the term *evidence-based* might be. And, when pushed, I did give my personal opinions to patients. But in general, I embraced the idea of providing patients with the best data that existed for interventions, such as mammography, colonoscopy, and prostate-specific antigen (PSA) testing, to help them make informed decisions. Similarly, I was much less likely than my father to recoil at the concept of guidelines, the algorithms provided by expert groups to help doctors manage complicated medical situations. In an era of rapidly expanding medical information and more sophisticated statistical analysis, it was wrong to assume that I knew best simply by dint of my personal experience.

And while I grumbled a great deal about Medicaid and HMOs, which forced me to make phone calls and write letters to get my patients various procedures, medications, or consultations with specialists, I appreciated why they were hassling me. The fact was that my father's generation of physicians, particularly after the passage of Medicare in 1965, embraced fee-for-service medicine with too much passion. Ordering tests was easy, and when the person or institution ordering them got paid to do so, there were no brakes on the system. Patients, too, reflexively assumed that more testing and treatment—regardless of the price—was better. The costs associated with health care had not been a major issue when my father began his practice in the early 1960s, but it had become an emergency when I began mine thirty years later, and Bill Clinton tried unsuccessfully to pass major reform legislation. So while I had no great love for insurance companies, I understood how physicians like myself needed help in determining which of our efforts were cost-effective.

I also rejected, to a large degree, my father's disdain for physicians who were willing to delegate patient care to their colleagues once they had left their offices or the hospital. This was, of course, tricky turf for me, as so much of my respect for my dad stemmed from his

utter devotion to his patients. But my sheer exhaustion during my
residency had opened my eyes to other models for covering one's
patients. Even my father, who had essentially lived in the hospital
during his training, characterized my internship as "absolutely ruthless and demanding." And, in retrospect, it had not been good for
him, my mother, my sister, and me that he had never found ways to
detach from his medical work, pursue other interests, and, potentially, reinvigorate himself. In some instances, perhaps, it might not
even have been good for his patients.

As of 1993, when I returned to Columbia, my general medicine
colleagues and I still followed our clinic patients when they required
hospitalization. But there was a new phenomenon on the horizon:
hospitalist medicine, a specialty made up of physicians who covered
other doctors' patients when they were in the hospital. Many of us
initially rejected this idea. After all, general internists strove to know
their patients inside and out and liked being in charge of their cases.
I could think of many instances in which I had discovered errors or
misperceptions in the care of hospitalized patients because I had
known them longer than anyone else involved.

But over the next decade, internists gradually began to admit our
patients to hospitalists. It made sense for a lot of reasons. Hospitalists not only were experts in in-patient medicine but knew how to
work the system to get patients expeditious and more cost-effective
care. Those of us who showed up in the hospital only periodically
were, frankly, lost at times.

The potential downsides of this new type of arrangement were
obvious. Concepts such as professionalism and humanism, which
medical schools and residency programs were increasingly empha-
sizing, had once been synonymous with total devotion to medicine and the care of patients. Now, patients were handed off from
doctor to doctor, not only from general internist to hospitalist but
from one hospitalist to another. Meanwhile, the house officers who
helped us care for patients had their own confusing schedules; their
chief residents sometimes even sent them home in the middle of the
day so they would not work too many hours. Care for their patients
could pass through several different doctors, including night floats,

before they returned the next day. Indeed, in 2013 a physician wrote an article praising one of her mentors, Joseph Lieber, who came to the hospital seven days a week, was a highly skilled diagnostician, and was "always nice" to his patients, and the *New Yorker* found it interesting enough to publish in its "Annals of Medicine" section.

Many physicians—not just old-timers like my father but some from my generation—bemoaned these new developments. One surgeon proudly recalled one of his mentors standing in the way of a resident trying to leave the hospital and telling him, "Once you lay your hands on a patient, that patient is yours." Another physician termed the eighty-hour workweek "pathetic, embarrassing, and paltry." "Calling," another wrote, "isn't a word you hear much anymore." Similarly, writing in 2002, a residency program director stated that limiting hours produced unsafe doctors. "Learning medicine," he wrote, "is different and requires physical effort that may seem inappropriate to those in other professions."

On rounds at Columbia, my longtime nephrologist colleague Jay Meltzer taught physical examination and differential diagnosis on each admitted patient in the thorough, even painstaking, style that he had been taught. But the Department of Medicine eventually informed Meltzer that he needed to speed things up. House officers had complained that he was picking up too many new findings on his examinations. "Unable to teach badly," Meltzer told me, "I had to resign." Meltzer's and my colleague cardiologist William P. Lovejoy was nearly apoplectic when he read an op-ed piece written by a physician in the *New York Times* stating that the only reason to do physical examinations was to provide patients with a "hands-on" feeling. "I can think of a thousand diagnoses she's missed," Lovejoy railed.

But much to the chagrin of these venerable physicians, this way of practicing and learning medicine has largely ended. Sad to say, physicians are much less likely now to spend time with patients, make provisional diagnoses, and then revisit those diagnoses as the clinical situation evolves. Rather, doctors now send patients for CT scans and MRIs that reveal the diseases in question. Many modern physicians now have tablet pockets sewn into their white coats to ensure easy access to their iPads on rounds. Nor is exhaustion on the wards a badge of honor. Physicians—both women and men—are eager to have outside interests and be more active parents than their predecessors were. When Meltzer retired in his eighties he wrote a heartfelt letter to his patients saying that medicine had structured his life "for daily learning and discovery," a goal that few modern physicians likely seek. Even Louis Weinstein's fabled Monday-evening journal club, which my father had so avidly attended during his years in Boston, could not survive in this new era. Weinstein's trainee and colleague Sherwood Gorbach tried to keep it going, but the infectious diseases fellows had rebelled at spending evenings away from home. Some of them even preferred to watch *Monday Night Football*!

As a historian of medicine and my father's son, I well understood the pull of this old model of medical practice. But I also sincerely believed that spending time away from the hospital potentially *enhanced* one's ability to be a skilled professional—by broadening one's horizons and lowering the likelihood of burnout. And, as I suggested to my students and residents, these new arrangements actually freed up some time that could be used to directly improve patient care. For example, my using the hospitalists' services did not prevent me from visiting my hospitalized patients. Even if I was no longer writing daily notes in their charts, I could speak with my patients, eyeball the situation, and, if necessary, provide some suggestions to the other doctors. These visits were analogous to the second looks that my father and Weinstein liked to make on their sickest patients before they left the hospital for the day. Extra time could also be spent phoning discharged patients at home to check on their progress and confirm follow-up appointments. Or doctors could promptly call outpatients with the results of major tests, so such individuals did not have to anxiously wait until their next appointment. The fact was that being a good doctor no longer necessarily meant knowing every last detail of patients' cases or completely understanding the biological basis of their diseases, but rather using one's training and skills to supervise their care and make sure that their basic wishes and goals were elicited and respected. Part of this effort, I had to admit, involved using UpToDate and other computer-based tools that provided quick and reliable information. Some might see this as cheating, but even my father, toward the end of his medical career, had thrown up his hands and admitted there was no other way an infectious diseases specialist could keep up with the expanding amount of knowledge within his own field, let alone in all of internal medicine. The days of his reading twelve weekly or monthly medical journals from cover to cover had ended.

Among the authors whose works my father read and admired was the writer and critic Anatole Broyard, who penned a series of essays about medicine after being diagnosed with terminal prostate cancer in 1989. Perhaps more so than any author, Broyard identified a series of qualities that made for a good doctor—even in a world of technological medicine and time constraints. Several of these reminded me of my dad. One was being a physician who viewed a serious illness as a crisis for the patient in question, not simply as a routine incident in his or her medical practice. Another quality was being a doctor who—even if only for five minutes at a time—would genuinely bond with patients, brooding on their situations and seeing the comedy and tragedy of their stories. These humble and perceptive insights are why I often assign a Broyard essay when I teach.

Of course, I still cringe at the notion of doctors doing shift work. I have encountered some physicians who, unfortunately, see their commitment as ending as soon as the clock says that it does. And I am well aware that fragmented patient care may lead to more medical errors, worse outcomes, or patient dissatisfaction. Fortunately, to this point, studies have not corroborated such concerns. Looking at house officers who are actually awake during noon conferences and seem relatively happy and well adjusted, I continue to believe that the changes have been for the best. And there remains, at least at the medical schools and hospitals where I have worked, evidence of great devotion and compassion. Perhaps this notion was best conveyed by an anonymous medical student responding to a surgeon's blog post that celebrated the days of the giants: "I am in medical school, and I could not imagine or design a class more full of energy or brilliance," the student wrote, pointing out that many of his classmates showed a special commitment to medicine, having started out in different careers and then spending years completing premedical work.

For me, a particularly vivid demonstration of commitment to patient care came in the wake of Hurricane Sandy in November 2011. I had just moved from Columbia University to New York University and the Bellevue Hospital Center in July. When Bellevue's patients needed to be evacuated after the storm damaged the electrical equipment, many of my new general medicine and primary-care colleagues stayed in the building for days, even carrying patients down darkened stairwells. When the hospital and its clinics remained closed, the Bellevue internists attempted to contact all of their clinic patients to see how they were faring and to get them medications and medical care. I cannot remember how many times I heard someone say, "These are our patients." It was inspiring and a throwback to my father's era, when house officers essentially lived in the "house."

Unfortunately for my father, things had continued to deteriorate at the Mount Sinai. In 1996, Primary Health Systems, a for-profit organization, purchased the hospital. Although my dad admitted that PHS had probably saved the hospital from total collapse, he believed that it made all decisions based only on costs. In 1997, the new administrators dismissed the chief of pharmacy in what my father termed a "ruthless" manner. Later that year, several neurologists and cardiologists, including my father's own cardiologist, defected to University Hospital. Members of the Mount Sinai's Infection Control Committee, which my father led, either resigned or were fired, leaving him as the only person on the committee.

In March 1998, things reached a crisis. The hospital's census and consultations were way down. Massive layoffs were planned for the next few weeks. Most worrisome, from my father's perspective, was a plan to change him and other full-time faculty members from a guaranteed salary to a stipend system, where doctors were paid per patient seen. Meanwhile, these physicians were still expected to teach for free. My father already believed that patient care at the hospital had sunk to an unacceptable level, and now it was sure to become worse.

"This is it," he wrote on March 28, 1998. "Push has come to shove!" His symptoms of anxiety and depression had increased, as had his baseline insomnia, heartburn, and vertigo. Plus, his misery was adding to my mother's burden of caring for Jessie.

"I see no other choice but to retire," wrote the man who had devoted his life to the practice of medicine and little else. He was not "emotionally ready for retirement" but it had been thrust upon him. "Now don't feel sorry for me," my father wrote to his imagined reader. He was only one of the many victims of the upheavals in medicine. My dad was especially grateful that all of this was happening when he was in his mid-sixties, nearing the end of his career. Younger physicians like me were not so lucky.

By April, my father had put a plan into place. On June 30, 1998, he would resign from the Mount Sinai Hospital. Fortunately, two infectious disease physicians from University Hospital had approached him about moving to their facility. Although he planned to do so, he would be acting mostly in a teaching capacity and not as a provider. "I've had it with patient care," he wrote. This decision made particular sense, as he had just reached two important milestones: it was forty years since his medical school graduation and twenty-five years since he had joined the staff of the Mount Sinai.

I was thrilled that the opportunity to move to University Hospital had arisen. I knew that my father was still an extremely talented physician and teacher who had an enormous amount to offer to patients and students. Plus, my mother was understandably dismayed at the notion of having my dad around the house all day. Aside from a brief interlude in which he had made sculptures from rocks, he had no hobbies. His life, he admitted, had been one of "fanatic involvement with medicine, my own field and medicine in general."

The last few weeks at the Mount Sinai were bittersweet. Several departments held farewell receptions in my father's honor and he received many good-bye notes. But he still felt very guilty about leaving. Luckily, my dad's associate, Cindy Gustaferro, joined a group of physicians who would cover the infectious diseases consultations at the hospital. On July 1, 1998, my father began what he called a "summer interlude," planning to assume his position at University Hospital in the fall.

When people asked my father whether he had left the Mount Sinai, he had a quick retort: "No, the Mount Sinai left me."

CHAPTER NINE

Slowing Down

Why was it taking my father so long to do everything? The two people who most studiously avoided answering this question were the two doctors: my father and me. Physicians are known for being the worst patients, and my father was no exception, attributing his symptoms to vertigo and problems with his balance. For my part, I did not want to know what I knew. As there were no treatments for early Parkinson's disease, what was the point of finding out?

But for anyone paying attention, it was pretty obvious that there was something wrong. My nonphysician wife, Cathy, for example, had good-naturedly nicknamed her father-in-law Slow-Motion Man. At the medical school, my dad had begun to give his lectures while sitting down. And, although the mental issues emerged after the physical problems, he was not as sharp as he once had been. Finally, in 2001, several years after his symptoms started, my father went to a neurologist and received a formal diagnosis of Parkinson's.

So imagine my surprise in 2004 when my dad casually mentioned that he was finishing up an article for the prestigious *New England Journal of Medicine*, the journal that had published his famous endo-carditis series in 1966. It so happened that I was completing a piece for the *New England Journal* at the same time and was working with the same editor. She was surprised—and pleased—to learn that we were father and son.

But that was my father's last hurrah in the world of medicine. As most Parkinson's patients do, he went into a steady decline. By

2007, he had stopped going to the hospital and medical school entirely, and then he gradually became homebound. In 2011, when he was seventy-nine, my mother finally had to put him in a nursing home, one that was affiliated with the facility of which he had been medical director over thirty years before.

My father was becoming the exact sort of patient who had once raised within him such concern and pity. Although I did so reluctantly, I gradually took charge of aspects of his medical care—just as he had done for my grandmothers. There was really no other choice. I was his son and a doctor. But what to do—and not do—for him could not have been more complicated.

Before his health deteriorated, my father spent some quality time at University Hospital. He was "not practicing medicine at the moment," he wrote in November 1999, but had "a professional address and identity." He taught medical students, residents, and fellows at the bedside and regularly attended conferences in the areas of infectious diseases and internal medicine. The hospital was always in need of excellent teachers, and his fellow faculty members loved having him around. My father was enormously appreciative of this opportunity and very fond of his colleagues, although he found his new institution to be "vast and impersonal" in contrast to the Mount Sinai.

He also became a bit of a gadfly at Case Western University School of Medicine's Department of Bioethics, attending its events and arranging for me to give an occasional symposium when I was visiting Cleveland. The faculty welcomed his involvement, although I had the sense that he used his medical degree to pull rank, foisting his impassioned beliefs about medical futility and other ethical issues on his new colleagues.

But medical reality was beginning to take over my father's life. When he finally saw the neurologist, he reported being unsteady and having difficulty getting out of low chairs. Buttoning his shirt was becoming hard. In addition, his voice had grown much softer, a condition known as hypophonia. There were occasional tremors—

involuntary movements of his arms. The neurologist confirmed these symptoms and found my father to be rigid with a stiff gait. "There are definite signs of parkinsonism," the doctor wrote. A second neurologist concurred: "We are most likely dealing with Parkinson's disease."

So how long had my dad been sick? His journals provide a clue. Almost three years earlier, on Wednesday, July 1, 1998, he penned an entry that became increasingly tiny and hard to decipher as he wrote. Micrographia—small writing—is another distinctive sign of Parkinson's.

His next note commented on the previous one. "The last note is *incredibly* sloppy and almost illegible," he wrote. "I wonder why?"

Even after receiving his diagnosis, my father could do very little about it. Generally, neurologists begin medications for Parkinson's only after patients' symptoms become debilitating, and my dad was still functioning pretty well. This is, of course, one of the reasons he had delayed obtaining a formal medical evaluation. In addition, my father was dealing with another medical problem, prostate cancer, which was discovered in May 2001 and treated by my sister's husband, Richard Stock, with a radium-seed implant in November of that year. Rich had actually thought that aggressive treatment was not necessary, but my dad had stubbornly insisted—another example of the perils of caring for a family member.

Once my father was formally diagnosed with Parkinson's, everyone knew what was coming. It was just a question of how rapidly the disease would progress and whether it would also affect his cognition. This inevitable decline is a major reason that my father's fellow infectious diseases physicians in Cleveland decided to honor him. Happily, they did so in a way that actually mattered to a man who cared little for awards. In early 2002, they formally named the citywide infectious diseases conference, which my dad had modeled on the conferences he had attended in Boston, after him. At one of these conferences, my father's junior colleague Robert Bonomo presented five cases, each one concerning an infection on which my father had published a landmark paper. It is hard to imagine better tributes to a colleague and mentor.

By the summer of 2002, my father's symptoms had worsened. "This is by way of announcing the momentous moment I first took medication for my PD," his July 31 journal entry read. Then, after almost falling on an escalator in January 2003, he added a second type of pill. In October of that year, he also went on Sinemet, the most common Parkinson's medication but one that neurologists avoid using until it is absolutely necessary. By early 2004, he was going into University Hospital less frequently due to a fear of falling. Eventually, my mother had to drive him there. Not surprisingly, my dad had to give up teaching in the infectious diseases committee—now called Mechanisms of Infection—for Case Western Reserve's second-year medical students. He had been the driving force for this teaching effort for at least twenty-five years.

Most worrisome were signs of mental slippage. As early as 1997, my mother had thought her husband was forgetting little things. Five years later, he confided in his journals that "I'm having trouble spelling certain common words." Soon thereafter, he reported a common side effect of Parkinson's medications: "hallucinations—visual—of a rather startling nature."

Then, in an entry dated January 29, 2004, my father wrote, "I'm even giving serious thoughts to writing one more medical paper." Had I read this note at that time, I would surely have been skeptical. After all, my dad's antibiotic manifesto was more than fifteen years overdue. He had not published a paper in eight years and, frankly, did not seem sharp enough to publish another one.

Yet somehow he pulled it off. And the story he chose to tell, in the August 5, 2004, issue of the *New England Journal of Medicine*, could not have been more fitting. It was about Leo Loewe, a physician at Brooklyn's Jewish Hospital who in 1942 had discovered that very high doses of the new wonder drug penicillin could cure previously untreatable alpha-hemolytic streptococcal endocarditis. But because it was wartime and there were shortages of penicillin, the US government had ordered that any available drug be sent for use in the military. Loewe, however, managed to forge a connection with a high-ranking executive at Pfizer, which was manufacturing the drug, even inviting the man to meet the endocarditis patients his company's drug had cured. As a result, the Pfizer executive quietly siphoned off penicillin and sent it to Loewe, enabling him to cure seven additional patients.

My father's essay was a sort of epitaph for his own career. In response to a letter sent to the *New England Journal* about his article, he admiringly termed Loewe a "desperate physician, eager to explore any avenue for his ill patient." For my father, there was no other way to practice medicine. But it was another example of changing ethical standards. These days, any sort of deception, even if done for the benefit of a patient, is frowned upon. And if sick patients were to learn that some of them were being deprived of a potentially helpful medication while others received it, they would loudly assert their rights. My dad appreciated these contradictions, admitting that "Loewe's heroics would not be possible today."

Even though my father stopped seeing his own patients after 1998, he still remained the unofficial physician for family and friends, as in the cases of Jessie and Gertie. This activity, something he called his "continental consulting service" in an April 2004 journal entry, persisted even after his Parkinson's was quite advanced. And I recall continuing to ask my father questions about complicated infectious diseases cases that I encountered. But as time went on and he realized that his advice might not be accurate, he was more likely to give inquiring relatives the names of other physicians that they might contact for formal second opinions. Still, my dad's expertise was so legendary that certain acquaintances, such as my parents' beloved next-door neighbors, continued to trust his judgment long after he shouldn't have been giving any opinions at all.

One of the most poignant aspects of my father's journals is how his growing difficulty in writing reflected the progression of his Parkinson's disease. By early 2000, less than two years after he had remarked on his sloppy note, his writing was routinely tiny, although, to his credit, still largely readable. On several occasions, he began notes by stating that he was going to make an extra effort to write in large print despite his micrographia. Inevitably, the size of the print shrank as the note progressed. It was a sad reminder of what a devastating disease he had. The notes continued into 2007, but they became increasingly short and unfocused.

My father's swan song came at my son's bar mitzvah, in February 2006. Phil was quite unsteady by this point and not traveling much at all. But getting to New York to share his grandson's big day was something he did not want to miss. When it was time for him to do an aliyah, a prayer uttered before and after a Torah reading, it seemed as if he would have to do it from his seat. But then my dad stood up and, with a shuffle, climbed the two steps to the platform, unsteadily but unassisted. On the return trip, he half raised his arms like Rocky, as if to say, *I did it!* On a day on which I recalled my own bar mitzvah and thought of all the relatives that I so dearly loved and missed, his presence—and his tenuous journey to stand next to his grandson—was profoundly moving.

Over the years, perhaps due to nostalgia, my father had become a little more receptive to Jewish rituals, including an occasional fast on Yom Kippur. And his love for family events and celebrations, even of a religious nature, remained strong. Although religion still meant little to him, his Jewishness was a constant. Ben's bar mitzvah, he wrote afterward in large print and capital letters, was "JOYFUL AND MEMORABLE." But by the time of my daughter Nina's bat mitzvah, in May 2008, he was too sick to travel, and my mother came by herself.

What followed was, as is routinely the case with Parkinson's disease, a slow but steady deterioration. For a couple of years, although my father was largely housebound, he could still walk up and down the stairs and, with great effort, go out to eat at a local restaurant. The situation was extraordinarily draining for my mother. Thanks largely to the spouses of people with Alzheimer's disease, the emotional travails of being a full-time caretaker have finally gotten proper attention. Parkinson's, although more a physical than a mental deterioration, raises the same issues of burnout. My mom, having just devoted years of her life to caring for her mother, now transferred her efforts to my father. As she was reluctant to allocate tasks to others, her burden was especially intense.

Eventually, however, she had to hire outside and then live-in help. By this point, it was quite clear that the Parkinson's was severely affecting my father's mental status as well, another common development. Although he could remember the name of the surgeon who had evaluated my grandfather Mannie's abdomen in 1975, my father did not recall that he had once been the medical director of the Montefiore Home. The visual hallucinations had gotten worse, requiring additional medications that made him groggy and caused him to speak a disquieting mix of fact and fiction. When my dad could no longer navigate the stairs, he was confined to the second floor of the house. It was a terrible state of affairs. In conjunction with my father's neurologist and me, my mother tinkered with his medications, but there was no real solution.

Right around Thanksgiving in 2011, a crisis occurred. The caregiver who was living at our house was away and my mother had broken her wrist. It was simply too much to keep my father at home. The time had come to send him to Menorah Park, a top-notch local nursing home. My sister and I flew to Cleveland to help with the transition. In retrospect, my mother had kept my dad at home far longer than anybody had thought she should. She felt bad about the transition, but my father did not. At this point, he was too confused to care where he was living.

My first image of my father sitting in the common room at the nursing home amid the other severely ill residents will always be lodged in my mind. He was in a wheelchair, sleeping, with his head hanging down. Many of the others looked the same. I vividly remembered similar assemblages of the infirm from my days volunteering at the Montefiore Home as a teenager. Then, my father was the supremely confident and able medical director, rushing around the building, caring for and reassuring such patients. Now he was one of them.

In some ways, Menorah Park staff members went out of their way to acknowledge who he was. They always called him Dr. Lerner and, at times, alluded to his expertise surrounding medical issues that arose at the nursing home. But in other ways, my mother felt, his status as a physician—a former leading light in the community—was insufficiently recognized. For example, it was hard to reach the nursing-home physician with questions. As there was not a neurologist on the staff, my mother had to track down the home's psychiatrist when she had questions about my father's Parkinson's medications. As a result, I found myself the frequent recipient of phone calls from my mom, asking for my opinion not only about his pills but also about his rashes, a new cough, or his bowels. Having now been drawn into the care of a sick relative myself, I found it harder to criticize my father for doing so.

My mother's frustrations extended beyond what went on at Menorah Park. She felt that my father's private neurologist was insufficiently attentive to him; he had told her that he could make recommendations only if my father could somehow get to his office. She also felt aggrieved at some of her own doctors. She was experiencing health problems herself and believed that, as in the old days, a physician's wife deserved a little extra attention. On a few occasions, staff members, rather than the doctors, called to give her the results of tests. Although I was able to help her interpret this information, she was offended that the doctors themselves had not phoned. After all of that professional courtesy my father had provided over the years, it was the least that these physicians could do. But as my dad knew better than anyone, that old-school type of medical practice was rapidly disappearing.

I tried to visit Cleveland as much as possible, but my family and job were in New York. Even though she was no longer his primary caretaker, my mother became a fixture in the nursing home, watching out for not only my father but the other residents. She knew my father had a gradually debilitating disease but remained engrossed in his day-to-day symptoms. During a particularly good stretch, she might call to say that my father was getting better. On a bad day, she would announce that he had taken a major turn for the worse.

As a doctor, I knew these were the ups and downs of Parkinson's, and, from five hundred miles away, I gently reminded her of this fact. She knew it too, of course, but it was understandably hard for her not to read too much into small things. Like other caring spouses, my mother fixated on minor issues in an attempt to retain some degree of control over such a disturbing situation. On several occasions, she asked my opinion about obviously nonsensical things that my father had said about his medical condition. When I asked her why she gave them any credence, she told me that she was so accustomed to my father being an authority on the family's health that it was hard for her not to still believe him. Fortunately, my uncle Allan was also a frequent presence at Menorah Park, keeping a close eye on his brother and the various medical issues that emerged.

One additional task remained. Now that my dad was in a nursing home, my mom and I needed to know what to do when his medical condition deteriorated. Would he go to a hospital? And, if he did, were there limits on what we would ask the doctors to do? I knew my father's mental condition was not great, but he did have moments of lucidity. It seemed logical to ask him what he would or would not want.

I knew what answer I wanted to hear, especially after reading my father's journals. I knew that he had devoted much of the later years of his career fiercely defending the right of people in situations like his to die with dignity, avoiding endless courses of antibiotics and other heroic technological efforts. I also knew that he had gone farther in certain cases, even speeding the dying process.

We had discussed this issue at length as recently as 2005, when the tragic Terri Schiavo case was finally coming to a close. Schiavo was a young woman who had suffered a cardiac arrest and massive brain damage in 1990, likely due to complications of bulimia. Schiavo's parents objected when, in 1998, her husband and legal guardian, Michael Schiavo, asked that doctors remove Terri's feeding tube and let her die. Robert and Mary Schindler believed that their daughter responded to them and might still improve, despite the fact that a CT scan of Terri's head showed minimal remaining brain tissue. After dozens of court hearings, Schiavo died on March 31, 2005, after her tube was finally permanently removed. My father, not surprisingly, had railed against the Schindlers and the pro-life activists and politicians who had rallied to their cause. Terri Schiavo's cardiac arrest had surely been a tragedy, but what her loved ones had done to her for fifteen years was, in his view, far more tragic.

Another piece of information was a document that I had found among my father's writings. Penned in February 2007, it was entitled "Epitaph," although he had had trouble spelling the word. He was, he wrote, in the "terminal phase of Parkinson's disease," losing the ability to both ambulate and control his bodily functions. His memory was "rapidly failing" him. After thanking my mother, his children, his grandchildren, his brother, his cousins, and his colleagues for all the blessings he had received throughout his life, he wrote that he was "taking steps to ease my passage." This was, of course, incredibly dangerous territory to begin with, and his growing inability to record coherent thoughts made it hard to understand what he wanted.

One thing was for sure. "Ronnie," he wrote, "doesn't deserve to struggle with me anymore." But how she would avoid this was not clear. At one point, for example, he wrote that he foresaw a "home hospice situation." But he also alluded to some type of suicide or euthanasia, noting that some in his situation "have taken drugs."

With all that I had learned, I wanted my father to passionately declare that his current condition—largely immobile, usually lethargic, and often confused—was unsatisfactory. But when I asked whether he would be willing to go to the hospital if he got sick, he said yes. And he even said that he would be willing to go on a ventilator.

"Sometimes they can really help," he told me, much to my disappointment. "It depends on what the infection is." He did say, in response to my prompts, that he would not want heroic treatment if it was clear that it would not work.

Then I asked if my dad if he was content with his current life, living in a nursing home with physical and mental limitations.

The man who had dreaded ever winding up like this answered, "Yes."

In retrospect, I might have raised these questions earlier in my dad's illness, when he was more mentally sharp, but, like my father and mother, I was to some degree in denial. So I had to use the information that I had.

What I had learned was especially compelling for two reasons. First, there is a common conundrum in bioethics in which patients who have fiercely favored a particular course of action over a prolonged period suddenly change their minds—often at a time of crisis. Just what were doctors supposed to do in this type of scenario? What were such patients' "true" wishes? What was my father's true wish? Even though I had hoped his beliefs would remain consistent, I knew that certain ethicists had convincingly argued that precommitment to a certain end-of-life strategy should not be inviolate. When experiencing something they had never previously encountered, people had the right to change their minds. So did my dad? My father's about-face was worrisome for another reason: it made me question the validity of his own assumptions about the inappropriateness of aggressive treatment for his severely ill patients and relatives.

Second, as I asked my father these questions, trying to figure out the right thing to do, I was—reluctantly, to be sure—becoming his doctor. Although I was glad to give friends and family members occasional medical advice and steer them toward my most trusted colleagues, I had carefully avoided replicating my father's decision to become actively involved in the care of relatives. But here I had no choice. Certainly no one at the nursing home was stepping up to the plate, aside from a nurse who had informed my mother about a hospice program. Now, along with my mom and sister, I was going to have to decide my father's medical fate. I suspected that he had felt a similar sense of obligation when confronted with relatives whose health was deteriorating.

Having been thrust into this role, and despite the valid objections to precommitment, I felt quite certain about what course of action was best. I believed to some degree that my father was happier in his current state than he would have anticipated. He was not in pain and still ate with gusto. He knew who we were and, at times, could engage in coherent discussions. But he spent most of the time either sleeping or drowsy, lacking the stamina to keep up a conversation. His quality of life was severely diminished. Ultimately, I concluded that it was impossible to advocate such specific choices so fervently in one's lifetime without them being a part of one's permanent makeup—even if they could no longer be articulated. My mother, sister, and uncle concurred with this assessment.

One of the many famous quotations that my father interspersed among his journal entries was one by the eighteenth-century English physician and intellectual Thomas Fuller about what constituted a good doctor. "When he can keep life no longer in," Fuller wrote, "he makes a fair and easy passage for it to go out."

I would be that good doctor. We put my father into Menorah Park's hospice program. Antibiotic pills at the nursing home were okay, but there would be no trips to the hospital, let alone ventilators or intensive care units, even if there was a hope that he could recover from a particular illness.

In October 2012, we all went to Cleveland to celebrate my father's eightieth birthday. I could not help but contrast this event with his own mother's eightieth birthday, twenty-three years before. On that day, dozens of relatives had attended the festivities at a country club. Pearl was in great physical and mental shape and had a wonderful time.

My father, in contrast, was going downhill. He could not really engage in meaningful discussions anymore. There were glimmers of his old self, as when he shooed me away, hugged my seventeen-year-old daughter, Nina, and tried to share with her some grandfatherly wisdom.

A couple of weeks later, I got a text from my sister. *Mom says Dad is not doing well*, it said.

At that moment, I was actually at a rescue shelter in the Bronx. It was a few days after Hurricane Sandy had ravaged the New York area, during the time that Bellevue was closed. I was tending to patients from a residential home who had been displaced by the storm.

I stepped outside and called the nursing home. The nurse told me that Allan was at the bedside.

"It's not good," he told me. Apparently there was a virus going around the nursing home. My father must have caught it and had possibly developed pneumonia. When his breathing became labored, the hospice team had given him morphine for comfort.

"He's not responsive," my uncle said. Six hours later, my father died.

The doctor in me knew this was for the best. His day-to-day existence had been terrible. We had all just visited and had the chance to say good-bye with many kisses, hugs, and loving words.

Yet I was not just a doctor but also a doctor's son. I thought to myself: *How could my father be felled by a nosocomial infection, the type of thing he routinely used to swat away as an infectious diseases expert?* It was the exact sort of story that my father and his colleagues had shared at medical meetings, recounting the sad, and at times ironic, fates of their brethren who had died of the exact diseases they had once conquered.

Finally, I was not just a doctor's son, but a son. As long as he was still capable of acts of warmth, especially to my children, how could we let him go? Despite her overall sadness and frustration with the situation, my mother had told me of occasional moments when my father was like his old self. When my uncle said my father was unresponsive, part of me had wanted to fly immediately to Cleveland and try to save him.

But when all was said and done, I thought of my father's patient Susan, who he somehow kept alive for years despite her leukemia and severe infections. He was upset at having been in France when she died but realized it may have been for the best. He was too involved in too many ways. Maybe the same was true for me.

We all flew into Cleveland, my family and my sister's family. There was no funeral and no shivah. He had told me dozens of times that these religious rituals were meaningless for him, and we honored his wishes. We instead held a non-shivah shivah at Allan's house, enabling family, friends, and my dad's colleagues to pay their respects. So many people present had relied on medical advice from my father over the years that it seemed illogical that they were still alive and he was not. Fortunately, I got to hear lots of wonderful stories about my dad as both a physician and a man. One relative gently grabbed me by the shoulders and insisted that I understand how he left no stone unturned in his devotion to her dying husband. "He practically lived at our house at the end," she told me.

But in a world dominated by the Internet, it is fitting that perhaps the best tribute could be found online, at a legacy site on which mourners can post comments. My favorite was from someone I had never met—a man in Texas—who wrote: "I was one of Dr. Lerner's last patients before he retired. His efforts, skill, devotion and tenacity are the reason that I am still alive today. Dr. Lerner never gave up on me and he saved my life. Not a day goes by that I do not think of him at some point."

Me too.

Epilogue

The ethical conflicts between my father and me, and between his generation of physicians and mine, are not merely of historical interest. On the one hand, most experts would agree that patient autonomy has triumphed over physician-based paternalism. One visit to a meeting of a hospital ethics committee or an institutional review board in charge of evaluating research protocols should demonstrate the primacy of informed consent. Nothing can be done to a patient or subject without his or her explicit approval. Similarly, thanks to the Internet, many patients and families dealing with complicated medical decisions at times know as much or more than their doctors. AIDS patients in the 1980s and 1990s were especially known for their expertise, but many modern cancer patients—and individuals with rare diseases—are equally knowledgeable. In addition, patients with terminal diseases have taken the initiative in setting limits to their treatment and, in certain states, can avail themselves of physician-assisted suicide.

On the other hand, as can be seen by the growing number of articles on the limits of autonomy and the myth of self-governance at a time of illness, the triumph of patients' rights has never really been complete. There are plenty of patients and families with little interest in making their own medical decisions. "What do you think I should do, Doctor?" is a common question in my office. In some instances, the ramifications of various choices are so genuinely complicated that it makes little sense to expect laypeople to know what should be done. Research has shown that the more options patients are given, the more likely they are to throw up their hands and ask the doctor what to do. Just as paternalism's historical moment came under fire, so, too, has the historical moment of pure autonomy.

Given these barriers to the autonomy model, some educators have promoted the idea of shared decision making, in which a health-care provider and a patient work together to review the scientific literature and the patient's preferences to reach decisions. A recent development in the field of shared decision making that would have been of great interest to my father is the Physician Orders for Life-Sustaining Treatment (POLST) form, in which, after discussions with a patient, a physician places an actual order in the medical chart specifying what types of medical care will be offered at the end of life.

It is hard to object to the concept of shared decision making. Indeed, it is more or less what I practice in my office, especially when dealing with complicated medical decisions such as cancer screening, in which the scientific literature gives conflicting recommendations. But I think my father would have argued that doctors can still do better.

As I learned from his journals, my dad practiced a style of medicine in which he immersed himself in both the medical and emotional aspects of the case. He not only knew the science but also had vast clinical experience, giving him information that one could not obtain from simply reading the results of randomized clinical trials. This is just the sort of knowledge that his never-published article on antibiotics would have stressed: giving only as much medication as was necessary, tailoring the antibiotic choice to the type and severity of the infection, distinguishing dangerous from benign bacteria, and, occasionally, withdrawing all antibiotics and letting the patient's immune system take over. Further, my father made a point of getting to know as much about his patients as he could, including their backgrounds, their beliefs, and their previous encounters with the medical system. He even agreed to be the repository for their anger and frustration—as long as they would then follow his advice. Armed with all this knowledge, making expert recommendations to his patients followed naturally, as did the patients' acceptance of his advice.

It is not as if my dad disregarded patients' wishes and simply told them what to do. To the contrary, he believed that it was his job to incorporate what he had learned about them into his ultimate medical recommendations. Interestingly, Dartmouth physician and researcher Albert G. Mulley Jr. has recently championed a similar concept in which doctors attempt to diagnose their patients' preferences, thereby leading to more accurate assessments of what patients really want. This, then, may be the ultimate goal of the therapeutic interaction: trying to arrive at the *best* choices for the patient—not merely the ones that empowered patients would choose on their own. Of course, having said this, it remains crucial not to silence patients or force choices onto them, two things done routinely in the era of paternalism.

Moreover, the time may be especially ripe for reviving the type of expert advice that my father sought to provide. We are gradually entering an era of what is being called personalized or individualized medicine. Traditionally, physicians have confronted disease by using blood tests, culture results, X-ray imaging, and tissue specimens to diagnose and then treat specific conditions. The new paradigm draws on the observation that diseases differ in different patients. For example, different breast cancers have different genetic patterns, and these patterns help to determine how aggressive the cancers are and which treatments will and will not be effective. Meanwhile, because of genetic variation between individuals, drugs that work for some people may not be good choices for others. To the degree that the information generated by personalized medicine is accurate, there may be fewer instances in which doctors and patients need to compare the risks and benefits of specific interventions. That is, there may be one best course of action that wise and compassionate physicians can guide their patients to take. The same type of personalized approach is applicable to controversial screening tests. For example, mammography may be more beneficial for certain patients than for others.

A second important development is the passage of the Afford-able Care Act, President Barack Obama's effort to expand health care coverage for Americans. A primary mechanism for accom-plishing this goal is to rein in spending, which has spiraled out of control. As of this writing, health care makes up over 17 percent of the US gross national product, but Americans do not have substan-tially better health outcomes than citizens in countries that spend considerably less. Roughly one-quarter of Medicare spending oc-curs during the final year of patients' lives, suggesting that expen-sive technologies are being used on elderly patients who will soon die anyway. Blame for the excessive spending can be directed at sev-eral factors: fee-for-service physicians who liberally and reflexively order tests and therapies that are of limited value; pharmaceutical and technology companies that aggressively promote their prod-ucts through direct-to-consumer advertising; and, more broadly, a culture that defies—rather than accepts—the inevitability of death. Also contributing are patients and families who automatically tell doctors to do everything when doing less would be appropriate. Perhaps the most famous patient in this regard was the writer Su-san Sontag, who, her son later wrote, would not hear that she was dying. Sontag essentially bullied her doctors into trying all con-ceivable therapies for her fatal leukemia, although the treatments only prolonged her suffering.

As health-care reform efforts proceed, there is a role for good doctors who strive to know the scientific literature and who use that knowledge to help patients appreciate the likely value of technologi-cal interventions in the context of their own specific cases. My father loved the challenge of choosing antibiotics and curing patients, but he vehemently opposed treating infection after infection in perenni-ally hospitalized demented patients with a poor quality of life—let alone allowing them to return to the intensive care unit or be placed on a breathing machine. My dad knew when to be aggressive and when it was smarter to pull back and stop the cycle of more and more testing—much like an experienced cardiologist might reassure a patient with a supposedly abnormal electrocardiogram that it is a normal variant, or a veteran neurologist might defer head scans when patients' headaches can be explained by doing a careful history and physical examination. This type of clinical judgment, which physician-writer Abraham Verghese and others have referred to as "bedside medicine" or the "art of medicine," seems especially important in an era in which the results of technological studies increasingly dictate physician behaviors and drive up costs.

What about death and dying in an era of health-care reform? The medical futility movement of the 1990s failed, in part, due to concerns that physicians like Phillip Lerner were championing the concept as a way to reassert their authority in managing death and dying. But my dad thought that judgments about futility emerged logically when knowledgeable and experienced physicians interacted with dying patients and their families in an intimate and ongoing manner. So it should come as no surprise that modern specialists in palliative care, who have expertise in assessing the physical and emotional costs of illness, have reinvigorated the futility debate in a way that emphasizes both their knowledge of the end-of-life literature and their hands-on approach to patient care. In a recent article in the *Journal of the American Medical Association*, for example, Columbia University palliative medicine specialist Craig D. Blinderman and colleagues proposed that instead of assuming CPR must always be offered, physicians should use a three-tiered approach when discussing its use with seriously ill patients: (1) consider CPR as a plausible option; (2) recommend against CPR; or (3) do not offer CPR. The hope is that this sort of framework can teach patients that resuscitation is not the choice in all cases but rather an option in those circumstances when it has a viable chance of being beneficial.

Of course, there are barriers to these efforts. One of these could not be more clearly demonstrated than in my father's case. Despite having a severely debilitating disease, my dad seemed content and even expressed a willingness to allow heroic technologies if they became necessary to save his life. That he had railed against this type of decision for years made his choice even more ironic. The fact remains that we are drawn to the use of antibiotics, respirators, and other interventions even when they may, at best, prolong suffering. In many cases, they even exacerbate it.

That is why it is good that palliative care and hospice teams now populate hospitals and nursing homes. Home hospice is another program that can address the complicated issues surrounding death and dying. Unfortunately, political opponents played on the public's fears and derailed the plan to fund discussions of end-of-life options through the Affordable Care Act, claiming that this effort would lead to the creation of "death panels," in which bureaucrats would supposedly use impersonal guidelines to unilaterally discontinue therapy. However, it is my experience that patients and families welcome thoughtful conversations about the limits of medicine with well-informed doctors who they trust. A 2013 survey by the Pew Research Center reported that two-thirds of Americans believe that there are circumstances in which doctors and nurses should allow patients to die. But such discussions should not necessarily end with the denial of aggressive treatments by physicians and insurers. Rather, the idea is to enable patients and families to understand the pros and cons of interventions from both a medical and a financial perspective.

Another important barrier to improving doctor-patient communication is inadequate time. Meaningful interactions and conversations may not occur because, more than ever, physicians face limits on how much time they can spend with patients. House officers who wish to stay late and talk with their patients are often sent home lest they accidentally spend too many hours in the hospital. An office-based practitioner is expected to see a new patient every fifteen to twenty minutes to compensate for low reimbursement rates. My father's work as an academic and a consultant with a minimal private practice allowed him the luxury of spending protracted amounts of time with patients. Fortunately, innovative team-based models for providing health care, such as the Patient Centered Medical Home, use computers, phone calls, and home visits to maximize the ability of physicians, physician assistants, nurse-practitioners, and clinical nurse specialists to use their skills most efficiently. The hope is that such models will give team members the time, when necessary, for more in-depth discussions about complicated medical issues.

Medicine today is a technological marvel. As I was writing this epilogue, I learned that scientists had discovered genetic patterns shared among patients with the most severe cases of breast, ovarian, and uterine cancers, raising the possibility of treatment breakthroughs for all three diseases. The New York Genome Center is conducting a research study in which full genomic sequencing of malignant glioblastomas will generate individualized treatment strategies for patients previously thought to all have the "same" disease. I also recently read that surgeons at the Children's Hospital of Illinois had inserted a tissue-engineered bio-artificial trachea in a two-year-old Korean girl born without a windpipe. Closer to home, my colleagues at New York University Langone Medical Center diagnosed a rare pancreatic cancer known as an insulinoma through elastography, a new technique in which a computer processes sound waves to produce images of tumors. Meanwhile, with respect to medical ethics, we have largely learned to do the right thing. Aside from occasional lapses, those scandals in which researchers, hospitals, or other representatives of the medical community run roughshod over the rights of patients or study subjects have largely disappeared. Ethics committees and institutional review boards are ubiquitous. The 2012 Sunshine Act requires online posting of all instances in which physicians receive anything more than trivial gifts from pharmaceutical companies or other commercial industries, making it easy to detect potential conflicts of interest. Finally, patients can access the Internet for information about standards of care, clinical trials, and new discoveries.

Yet in making all of this progress, we have lost something. The emphasis in the doctor-patient relationship has shifted from physicians getting to know patients and their illnesses to physicians doing things for patients and their illnesses. Most internists are actually quite adept at discussing the risks and benefits of mammograms, colonoscopies, and cholesterol pills, as well as the importance of DNR and consent forms, but not so good at just sitting and talking about how things are going. For several decades, using the skills he had learned from his mentors and the wisdom he had learned from his patients, my father was able to balance science, ethics, and humanism. It is my hope that this book will encourage current and future practitioners to do the same.

One of the many books I read while working on this project was *The Healer's Tale*, by the anthropologist Sharon R. Kaufman. Kaufman tells the stories of seven prominent twentieth-century American physicians who embodied humanistic, patient-centered medicine. They had all learned their craft in the 1920s and 1930s, when therapeutic options were limited but "medicine could be characterized by its sense of duty, charity and social obligation." Morality, Kaufman wrote, was thought to be "inherent in the practice of medicine itself."

I was especially interested to learn that four of Kaufman's subjects had been the children of physicians who had emphasized duty and caring in both their work and lives. The other three grew up with parents who, while not doctors, were humanitarians who served their local communities in a wide array of volunteer projects.

At this point, you might be wondering if either of Cathy and my college-age children, Ben and Nina, are planning to become physicians and if there will ever be a book about another generation of Dr. Lerners. The answer, at least for now, is no. Nor are they planning to follow their mother into the legal profession. Although I am thrilled to be a physician and would have been happy if one or both of them had wanted to follow in my footsteps, it would never have occurred to me to expect this or pressure them to do so. I don't recall ever bringing them with me to hang out on the wards when I made weekend rounds. Although I did discover a touching journal note in which my father announced his plans to send medical books to a nineteen-year-old premed granddaughter of one of his cousins, even he, when still mentally sharp, did not urge my kids to pursue medicine. While he still loved the career he had chosen, perhaps too much had changed.

I would be the last person to suggest that being the child of a physician makes someone a better doctor. But growing up with my father, I learned about the interrelationship of family, morality, and medicine. Doing the right thing mattered in the hospital and at home. My mother's illness and subsequent volunteer work only strengthened my convictions. Through my care of patients, teaching, and writing, I have, in my own way, tried to underscore how medicine—as much as any career—provides an opportunity to do good for vulnerable people. It is a privilege that I will always cherish.

Acknowledgments

Writing acknowledgments for an autobiographical book was particularly difficult, as I was tempted to thank everyone who has ever done me a good turn, something that is clearly impossible. So while I will formally acknowledge only some people, there are many more of you whose efforts over the years I appreciate.

The present task was made additionally difficult by the fact that one blogger called the acknowledgments in my previous book, *One for the Road*, "quite possibly the best I have read." As for the book itself, she wrote, "it was a wash," with a "preachy tone" that undermined my arguments. Well, I guess so. But with respect to the acknowledgments, at least, I have large shoes to fill, even if they are my own.

So here goes. My first thanks go to my parents, who are baldly on display throughout this book. When my father learned that I was planning to use his personal journals to tell his story, he was entirely thrilled, even though he knew that I would reveal some of his less admirable characteristics and decisions. He did not attempt to micromanage my writing at all. Nor did my mother, a quite private person. I know it was not easy for her to read about her own experience with breast cancer in the 1970s or her mother's deteriorating health and difficult death two decades later. But showing the same confidence in me that she has for over fifty years, she trusted my judgment.

My wife, Cathy, and my sister, Dana, read the manuscript in its entirety and made very helpful comments. It was interesting to see how we remembered certain events quite differently. I tried as best as I could to respect their memories, screaming, "Get lost! It's my book and not yours!" only a few times. My father's brother, Allan, was also of great help, providing several key recollections. My good friend Tom Frieden, who I first met in medical school and who also had a physician father, made numerous incisive comments on the manuscript. I benefited from presenting a talk based on the book at the Breslau Family Lecture in Baltimore in March 2013. My thanks to Erica Breslau for the invitation. Lee Breslau, my college roommate, was kind enough to remind me of the time my father lost his temper at a restaurant where we had had horrible service. When my dad loudly announced, "I am leaving now!" and started counting to ten, the waiter finally brought the check.

Cathy's and my children, Ben and Nina, loved their grandfather Phil, known to them as Paw, very much. I am glad that they and their cousin Gianna will have this book as one way to remember him.

Family and friends too numerous to mention have listened patiently and responded enthusiastically when hearing about my father and this project. Some of you may even be having nightmares about having to look at yet another possible book cover! Special thanks go to my mother-in-law, Ellen Seibel, and our longtime nanny, Margaret Frempong, who both always asked about my father when we returned from a visit to Cleveland. Seth Godin and Micah Sifry have patiently answered my embarrassingly jejune questions about blogging and marketing. And of course I need to thank our dog, Akeela, who kept me company as I was writing, asking only for occasional treats in return. Okay, not so occasional. But what a good girl.

In the course of writing this book, I talked to many helpful people about what it means to be a doctor, about the field of bioethics, and about my father. They include William Lovejoy, John Loeb, Jay Meltzer, Daniel Callahan, Willard Gaylin, Arthur Zitrin, Sherwood Gorbach, Larry Altman, Allan Weinstein, Ethel Weinstein, Keith Armitage, Robert Salata, Martha Salata, Robert Bonomo, Walt Tomford, Bob Kalayjian, Michael Lederman, Steve Gordon, Marty and Pat McHenry, Bob and Vincetta Dooner, Cindy Gustaferro, and Sam Miller. Sam, whose life my father saved, was generous enough to endow a lecture series in my father's memory. I also benefited by reading the manuscripts of new books by Naomi Rogers on the polio nurse Sister Kenny and by Gary Belkin on brain death.

My work colleagues have provided great support for me, both logistically and psychologically. There are many people I would like to thank at Columbia, where this book had its genesis. They include Ken Prager, Don Kornfeld, Ruth Fischbach, David Rosner, Ron Bayer, Amy Fairchild, James Colgrove, NiTanya Nedd, Steve Shea, and Rita Charon, as well as the rest of my former colleagues on the New York Presbyterian/Columbia Ethics Committee and in the Center for the History and Ethics of Public Health and the Division of General Medicine. Also, it was at Columbia where I first worked with the Arnold P. Gold Foundation, which generously made me one of its first Gold Professors at the time when I was starting my career. I would be remiss in not thanking the Robert Wood Johnson and Greenwall Foundations and the Johns Hopkins University Press, all of which have fostered my scholarship.

My new colleagues at New York University have been terrific. Special thanks go to my generous fellow physician-writer Danielle Ofri, who helped connect me with her editor at Beacon Press, Helene Atwan. Andrew Wallach, Marc Gourevitch, Sandy Zabar, Doug Bails, Barbara Porter, Art Caplan, Allen Keller, Cheryl Healton, Arthur Zitrin, and Leonore Tiefer provided support during an unexpected crisis. Thanks also to Bob Anderson, Stacy Bodziak, David Oshinsky, Jessica Wico, and Marty Blaser. The general medicine clinic at Bellevue is an inspiring place to practice medicine and filled with real professionals. There are simply too many to name.

Speaking of Helene, she is a great editor. Perhaps the best compliment about her came from my agent, Robert Shepard, who, after reading Helene's first set of edits, told me: "This is the way it was once done, and I'm thrilled to see that someone is still doing it." In addition to being a top-notch agent, Robert is also a first-rate editor himself. I should know. He liberally marked up my articles at the *Daily Pennsylvanian* thirty years ago. I have also greatly enjoyed working with the rest of the folks at Beacon, including Crystal Paul, Alice Li, Tom Hallock, Pamela MacColl, Susan Lumenello, and

Marcy Barnes. Tracy Roe did an expert job of copyediting and may have set a Guinness world record by removing the word *also* three times in a single paragraph.

Another group of people deserving recognition is the editors of the online blogs that publish my essays on history and medicine. They include Tara Parker-Pope, Toby Bilanow, and Michael Mason at the *New York Times* and Jim Hamblin at theatlantic.com. Finally, I would like to thank my colleagues at the American Association for the History of Medicine, which has been my main academic home for almost twenty-five years. I can't imagine a smarter, more collegial group of individuals. It is a huge honor for me to be delivering the AAHM's 2014 Fielding Garrison Lecture, which builds on this book.

Okay, so these weren't such spectacular acknowledgments. But I loved writing them.

Bibliographic Note

This book builds on the work on many talented physician-writers. Like lots of physicians in training, I read the memoir *The Doctor Stories*, a compilation of stories by William Carlos Williams, the New Jersey general practitioner and author who famously used to write poems on his prescription pads between patient visits. To Williams's credit, he never romanticized his struggles in caring for poor, immigrant families.

The next memoirist I encountered was Yale surgeon Richard Selzer, whose books of short vignettes, including *Confessions of a Knife* and *Letters to a Young Doctor*, I have often used when teaching. Medical students need only read "Imelda," the tragic story of a surgeon's altruistic act gone wrong, to learn an abiding lesson in humility.

I also discovered the works of another Yale surgeon, Sherwin Nuland. In contrast to Williams and Selzer, Nuland wrote about the history of medicine, not his own patients. While perhaps exemplifying the sort of Whig history that has gone out of fashion, his 1988 book *Doctors: The Biography of Medicine* beautifully exemplifies how proud my father's generation of physicians was of its forefathers. So does Michael Bliss's biography of the legendary doctor William Osler, published in 1999. But it was *Lost in America*, Nuland's moving 2003 memoir about his nonphysician immigrant father, that encouraged me to write a biography of my own dad.

Following the 1978 publication of *The House of God*, pseudonymous author Samuel Shem's fictionalized account of his internship, physician memoirs became a sort of cottage industry. Many deal specifically with medical school or residency training—crucial, and often tumultuous, periods in a physician's career. Others use stories of past patients to illuminate the challenges of patient care, often among disadvantaged populations. I am fortunate to have many excellent physician-writers as colleagues at New York University: Perri Klass, Danielle Ofri, Jerome Lowenstein, Gerald Weissmann, Eric Manheimer, and Oliver Sacks. I also want to give a special shout-out to my fellow Clevelander David Hellerstein and his wonderful 1994 memoir *A Family of Doctors*, which is perhaps the book closest to this one in terms of style and content.

Other physician-writers whose works I reread in preparation for this book include Jerome Groopman, Atul Gawande, Abraham Verghese, Sandeep Jauhar, Pauline Chen, Siddhartha Mukherjee, Robert Klitzman, and Melvin Konner. I recommend them all. Gawande's *Complications* is especially helpful for capturing the ethical issues that arise during medical training. Many of my fellow residents and I read Konner's *Becoming a Doctor*, written by an anthropologist who attended medical school, when it was first published, in 1988. I also recommend the essays of Abigail Zuger, a physician-writer whose work most often appears in the *New York Times*.

I am lucky to be part of a small but talented community of physician-historians. While most of the work we do is pure history, some of us also draw on our own clinical experiences to inform our historical work (and vice versa). Fortunately, my colleague Jacalyn Duffin got many of us to contribute to the wonderful essays in the 2005 book *Clio in the Clinic*.

Speaking of Duffin, I am often asked to recommend a quick book on the history of medicine for health professionals or other nonhistorians. Duffin's *History of Medicine: A Scandalously Short Introduction* ably fits the bill. So do William Bynum's *The History of Medicine: A Very Short Introduction*, Ira Rutkow's *Seeking the Cure: A History of Medicine in America*, and Gerald Grob's *The Deadly Truth: A History of Disease in America*. With respect to medical historiography—which is the history of the history of medicine—see Beth Linker's 2007 essay "Resuscitating the 'Great Doctor': The Career of Biography in Medical History" for the short version, and Frank Huisman and John Harley Warner's 2006 book *Locating Medical History: The Stories and Their Meanings* for the long version. On the history of bioethics, two of the books I mention in *The Good Doctor*, David Rothman's 1991 *Strangers at the Bedside* and Albert Jonsen's 1998 *The Birth of Bioethics*, still stand the test of time. For a more recent version of the story, try Daniel Callahan's modest and informative 2012 memoir *In Search of the Good: A Life in Bioethics.*

Good historians pay close attention to their primary sources, using them to write original articles and books while also scrutinizing their validity. That is, interviews, correspondence, and—especially for this book—journal entries do not necessarily provide straightforward accounts of past events. But in order to write an accessible narrative I have, in many instances, taken these sources at face value. Nevertheless, I realize that words written by or spoken about my father may represent what the historian Jeremy D. Popkin has called "elaborate authorial strategies" and thus may give a "distorted" record of events. So, too, I made very specific choices about which events to include and which to omit in the autobiographical portions of this book. For more on these topics, see Popkin's 2005 book *History, Historians, and Autobiography*, the historian David Lowenthal's 1985 book *The Past Is a Foreign Country*, Philip Roth's clever autobiography *The Facts*, and historian of medicine Nancy Tomes's insightful essay "Oral History in the History of Medicine" in the 1991 *Journal of American History*.